Techniques in Cardiopulmonary Physiotherapy

Subin Solomen
BPT, MPT (Manipal) CRD
Professor, EMS Memorial Co-operative Hospital and Research Centre
Perinthalmanna, Kerala

Pravin Aaron
BPT, MPT (Manipal) CRD
DPT, Loma Linda University, California, USA
Professor and Principal
Padmashree Institute of Physiotherapy
Bangalore, Karnataka

PEEPEE
PUBLISHERS AND DISTRIBUTORS (P) LTD.®

Techniques in Cardiopulmonary Physiotherapy

Published by
Pawaninder P. Vij and Anupam Vij

Peepee Publishers and Distributors (P) Ltd.
Head Office: 160, Shakti Vihar, Pitam Pura
Delhi-110 034 (India)

Correspondence Address:

7/31, First Floor, Ansari Road, Daryaganj
New Delhi-110002 (India)

Ph: 65195868, 23246245, 9811156083

e-mail: peepee160@yahoo.co.in

e-mail: peepee160@gmail.com

www.peepeepub.com

First Edition: **2018**
Reprint: 2020, 2025

ISBN: 978-81-8445-233-4

Dedicated to

My Parents, SV Solomen and Premila Solomen, My Wife Divya

And to My Children, Angelina and Jerome

– Prof. Subin Solomen

Dedicated to

My Students

– Prof. Pravin Aaron

Foreword

I am extremely happy to write the foreword for this exceptional book on **Techniques in Cardiopulmonary Physiotherapy**, which will be of great help to the students, teachers and practising Physiotherapists. Cardiopulmonary Physiotherapy is a specialized field in physiotherapy, where student need adequate reference materials. This book describes the various techniques adopted in cardiopulmonary physiotherapy practice. It will provide them with a framework to teach, learn and practice.

Prof. Pravin Aaron and Prof. Subin Solomen are associated with Padmashree Institute of Physiotherapy since many years. As educators, they have set standards of distinction in teaching. I praise for this commendable contribution, which has come at a time, university across the country are deciding to streamline the curriculum.

The book certainly conveys the understanding of the authors as teachers of the subject as this is reflected in the depth of the information given in the book.

Dr. Vasudeva R
Director
Padmashree Group of Institutions
Bangalore

Preface

The book titled **"Techniques in Cardiopulmonary Physiotherapy"** which is intended to cover all the principles and techniques used in cardiorespiratory conditions. The book has been compiled and made as per the curriculum according to the draft "Model curriculum handbook–Physiotherapy" prepared by Allied Health Section, Ministry of Health and Family Welfare (2015-16). The syllabuses of Cardiopulmonary Physiotherapy in different universities in India and abroad were also taken into consideration while writing this book. The audience for this textbook series are under graduates, postgraduates, clinicians and academicians in the field of physiotherapy.

In this book it is divided into 31 chapters. Chapter 1 scope of cardiopulmonary techniques in different conditions, look into the problem list of cardiorespiratory patient, identifies the short-term and long-term goals. Chapter 2-4 details the mechanism of lung expansion therapy, airway clearance techniques and reducing work of breathing in a cardio-pulmonary patient. Chapter 5-31 covers all techniques used in cardiopulmonary physiotherapy such as Neurophysiological facilitation of Respiration, Breathing techniques, Incentive spirometry, Mechanical aids in to increase lung volume and to reduce work of breathing, Positive pressure adjuncts, Coughing techniques, Postural drainage therapy, Chest manipulations, Suctioning, Autogenic drainage, Active Cycle Breathing Technique, Manual Hyperinflation, Other airway clearance techniques, Hydration and Humidification, Nebuliser, Medical gas therapy, Energy conservation and work simplification, Controlled mobilisation, Exercise prescription, Manual therapy in cardiorespiratory conditions, Chest mobility exercises, Relaxation techniques, Electrotherapy in cardiorespiratory disorders, Patient education, Complimentary therapy and Nutrition. Each technique is detailed in simple manner.

In the appendix several schematic diagrams were drawn which may help the students for their examinations. I hope my hard work will give noteworthy contribution to the teachers and students. Any suggestions or corrections are most welcomed and can be mailed me at *subins2001@rediffmail.com.*

Prof. Subin Solomen

Acknowledgements

First and foremost I would like to thank almighty God without whose blessing this book would have not been possible. I am sincerely obliged to Prof. Pravin Aaron, Principal, Padmashree Institute of Physiotherapy, who is also the second author of this book. He helped me in reviewing and correcting the script of this book. It was impossible to deliver this book without him.

I am indebted to my Principal Jinson K Paul, Dr. A Mohammed, Chairman, Sri M Abdunnasir, General Manager of EMS Cooperative Hospital and Research Centre, Perinthalmanna, Kerala for providing me support for writing this book. I am indebted to TK Narayanappa, Chairman, Dr. CN Ashwath Narayan, Managing Trustee, Dr. Vasudeva Director, and Prof. Rajesh Shenoy, Director of Padmashree Group of Institutions, Bangalore where I did my graduation and worked as lecturer to professor for their support and cooperation in writing this book.

I am thankful to Chairman, Managing Director and whole team members of Peepee Publishers and Distributors for publishing the book in a nice manner. I have taken lot of information from the books and articles published on physiotherapy techniques in cardiopulmonary disorders which I have mentioned in the last as "list of references". I acknowledge all the authors written on topics of cardiorespiratory physiotherapy both published and unpublished as I have borrowed information and ideas from these books and articles.

I especially thank Professor Pearlson Manual Therapist (FIMT) Padmashree Institute of Physiotherapy, for his contribution on chapter and photographs of the chapter titled Manual Therapy in Cardiorespiratory Conditions. I also thank Professor Prem Kumar, Mr. Sreejith, Mr. Chacko P George faculty and Mr. Naseef and Mr. Riyas students of EMS Cooperative Hospital and Research Centre, Perinthalmanna for helping me to make schematic diagrams.

My thanks also go to my students Mrs. Trupti, Mrs. Barnali, Mrs. Sumana Baidya, Mr. Vikram, Mr. Deepak Joshi, Ms. Sakuna, who all helped me in completing the book in the desired format. My thanks go to my wife Divya who has continuously encouraged and supported me in writing and completion of the book for the last three years.

Prof. Subin Solomen

Contents

Plate–I

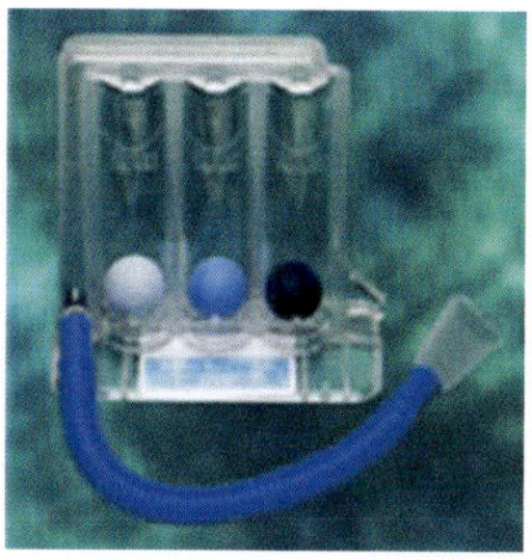

Fig. 8.1: Flow oriented spirometer: Triflo meter
(See page no. 31)

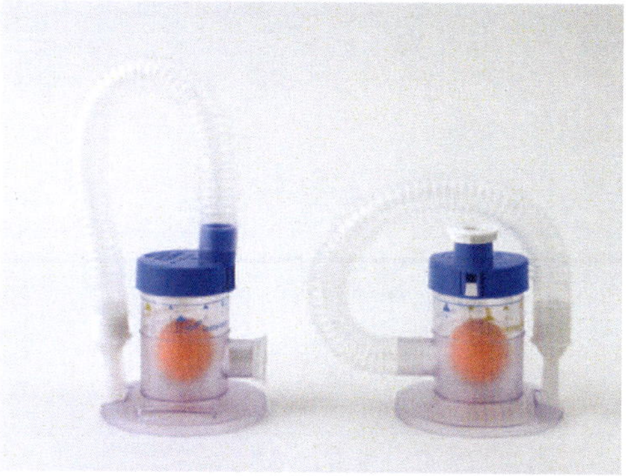

Fig. 8.2: Flow oriented spirometer: Mediflo
(See page no. 32)

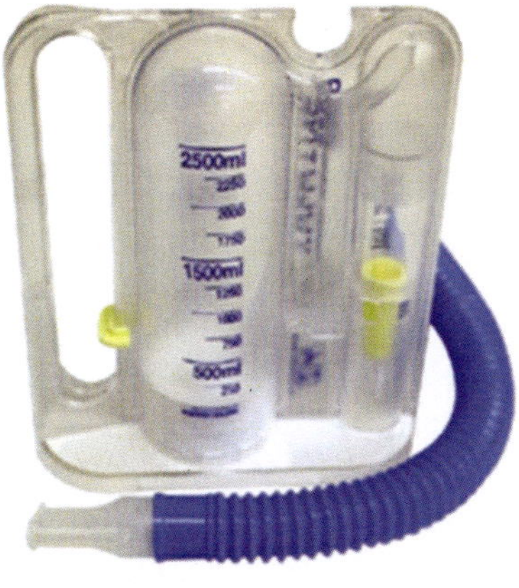

Fig. 8.3: Volume oriented spirometer:
Volydyne 2500 ml capacity (See page no. 32)

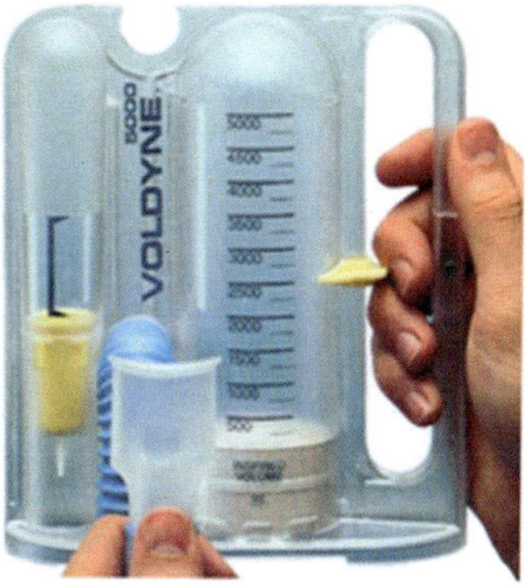

Fig. 8.4: Volume oriented spirometer:
Volydyne 5000 ml capacity (See page no. 32)

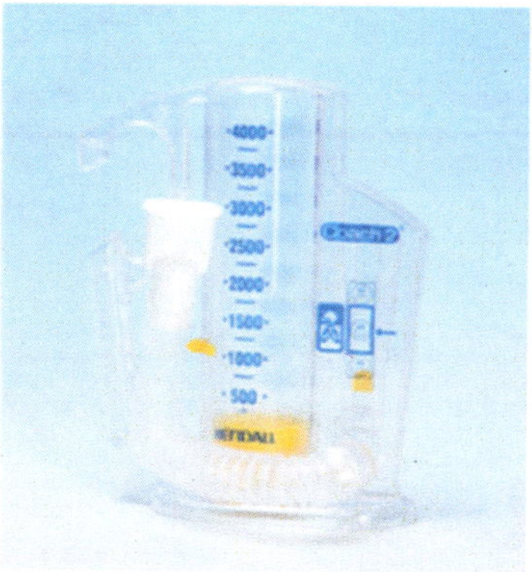

Fig. 8.5: Volume oriented spirometer: Coach spirometer
(See page no. 32)

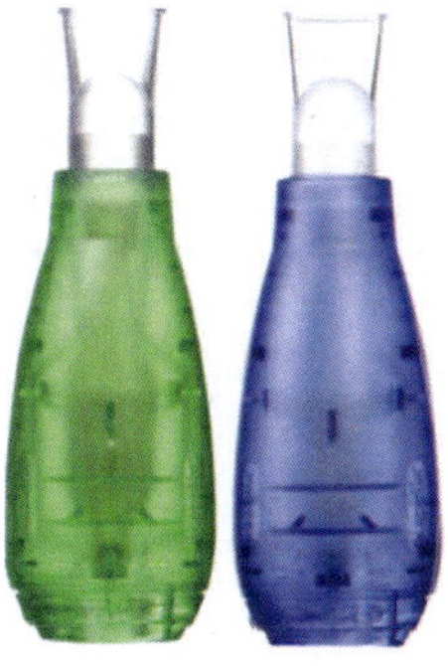

Fig. 10.5: Acapella (See page no. 41)

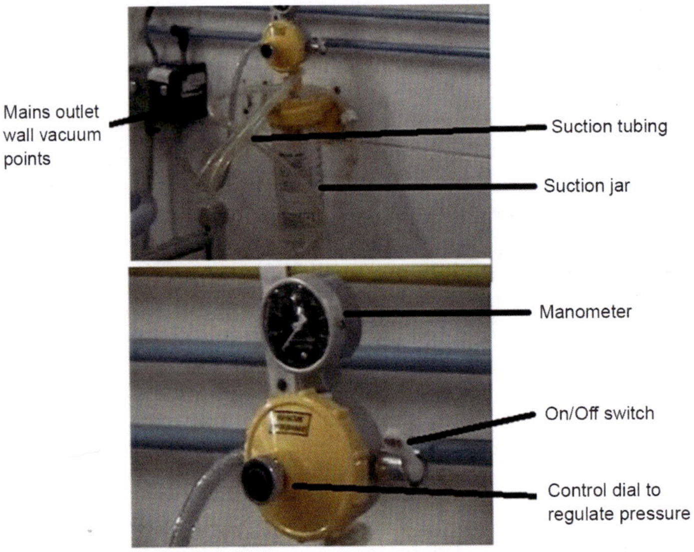

Fig. 14.4: Parts of central suction apparatus (See page no. 59)

Size in FG	Colour	Plain	Thumb Control	Finger Tip Control
5	Grey			
6	Light Green			
8	Blue			
10	Black			
12	White			
14	Green			
16	Orange			
18	Red			
20	Yellow			
22	Violet			
24	Light Blue			

Fig. 14.7A: Suction catheter of different size with color code (See page no. 60)

Plate–III

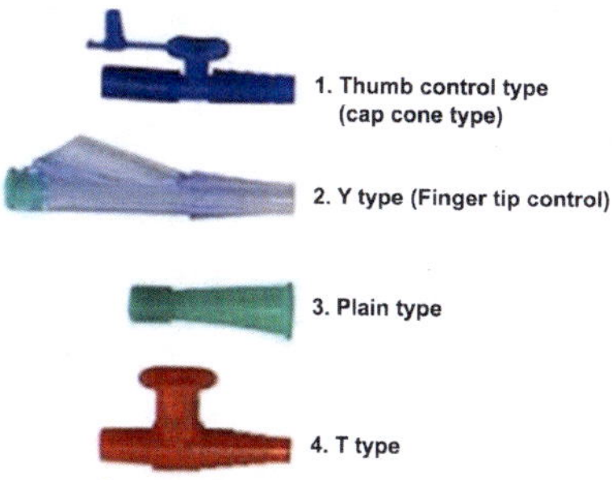

Fig. 14.7B (See page no. 61)

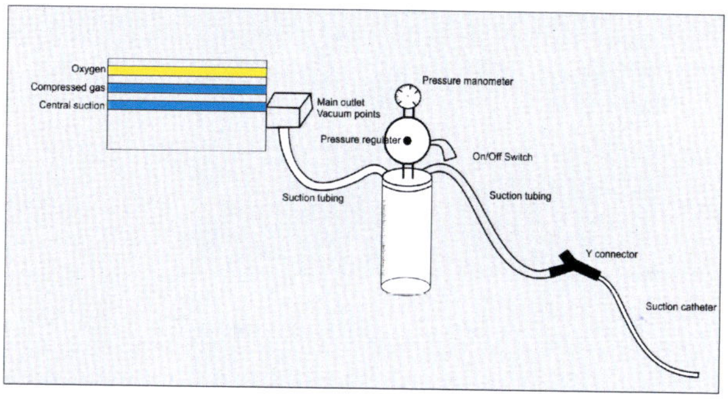

(See page no. 145)

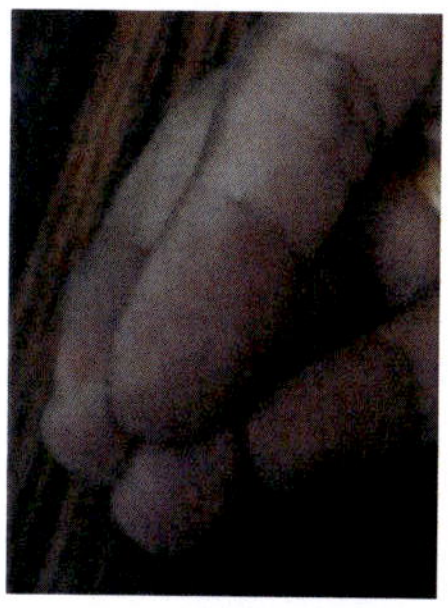

(See page no. 142)

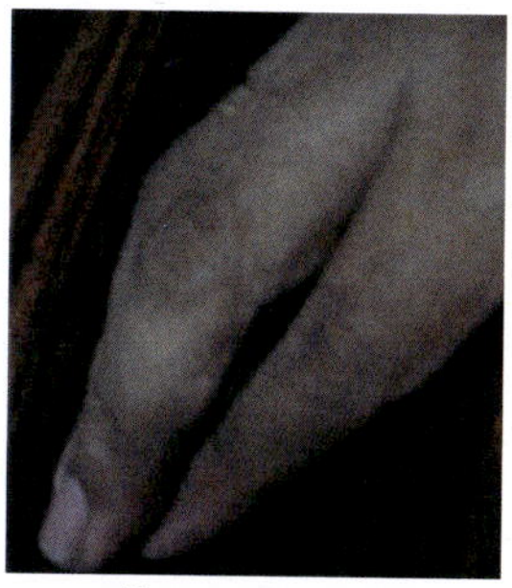

(See page no. 142)

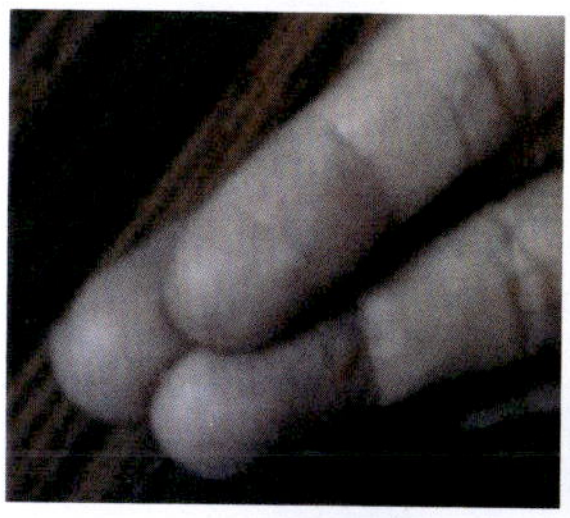

(See page no. 142)

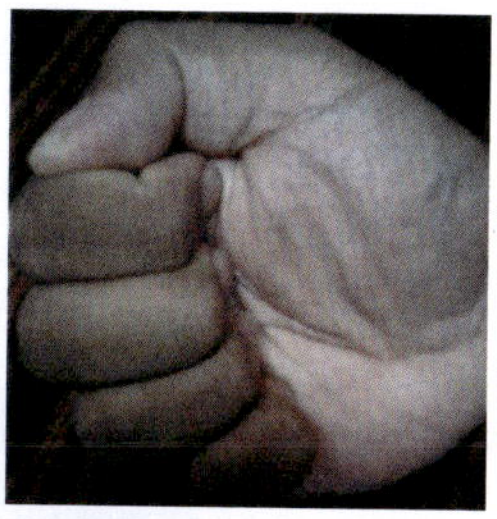

(See page no. 142)

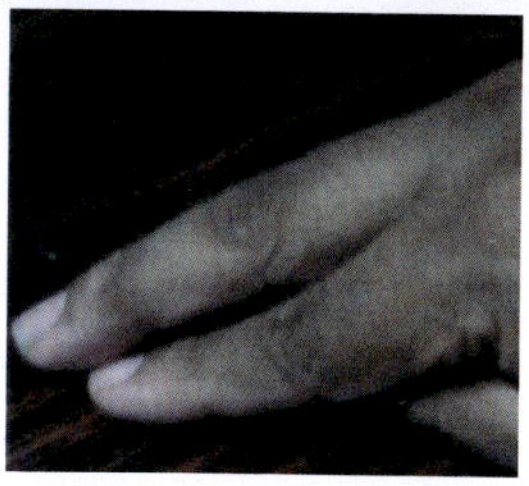

(See page no. 142)

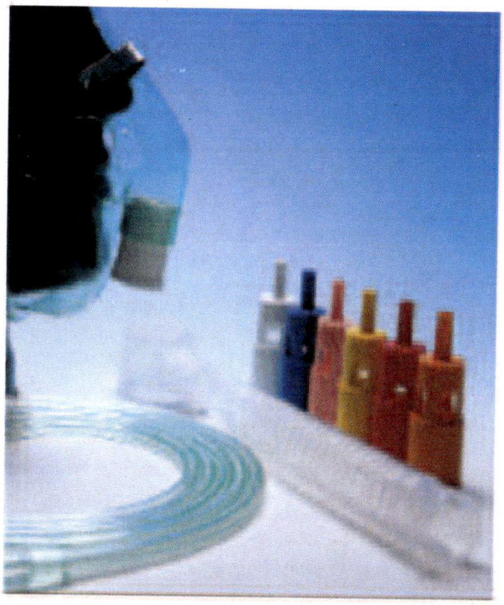

Fig. 21.10: Jet nozzle and entrainment ports
(See page no. 92)

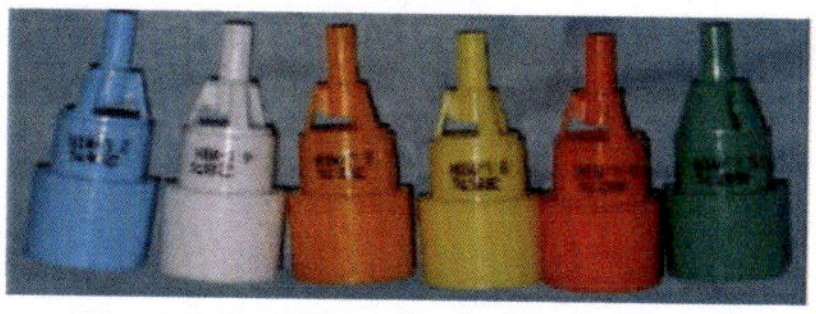

Fig. 21.11: Different entrainment port
(See page no. 92)

IV—Plate

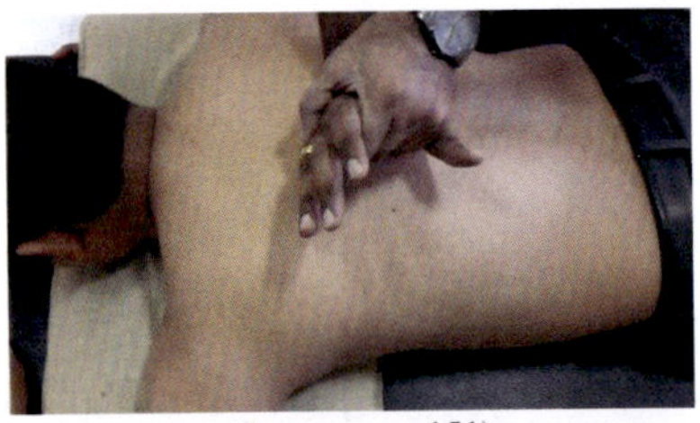
(See page no. 151)

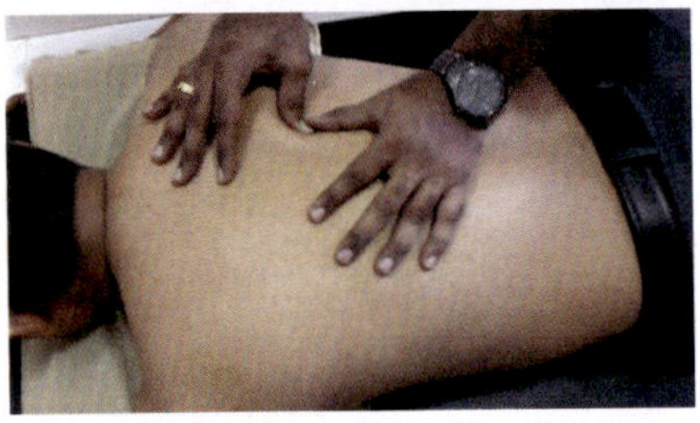
(See page no. 151)

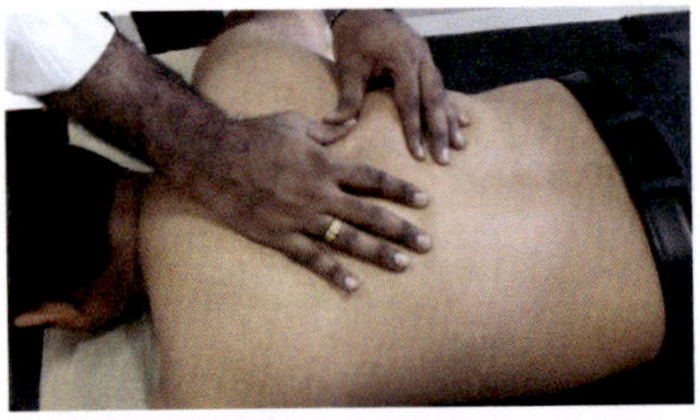
(See page no. 151)

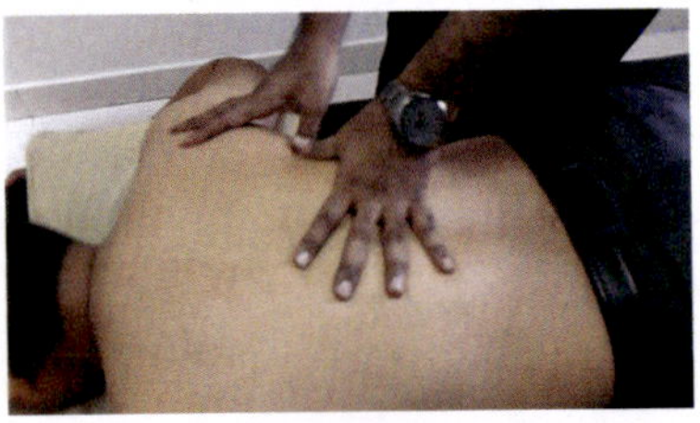
(See page no. 151)

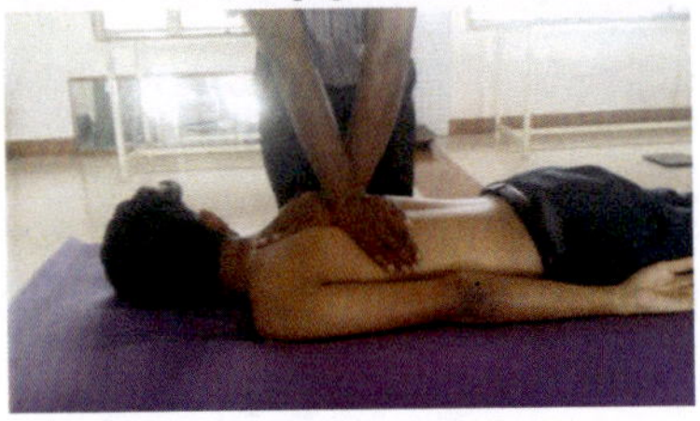
(See page no. 151)

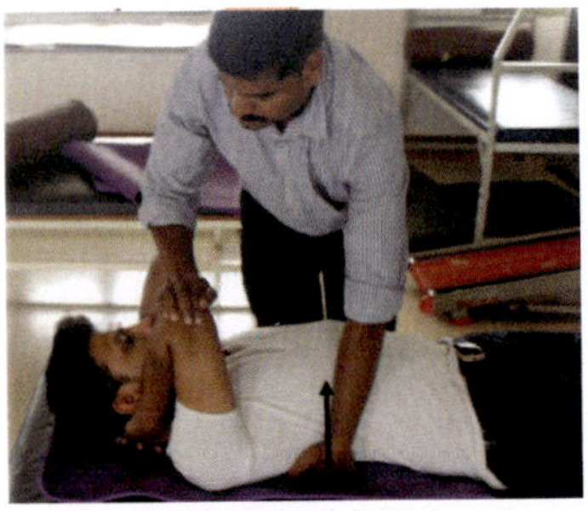
(See page no. 152)

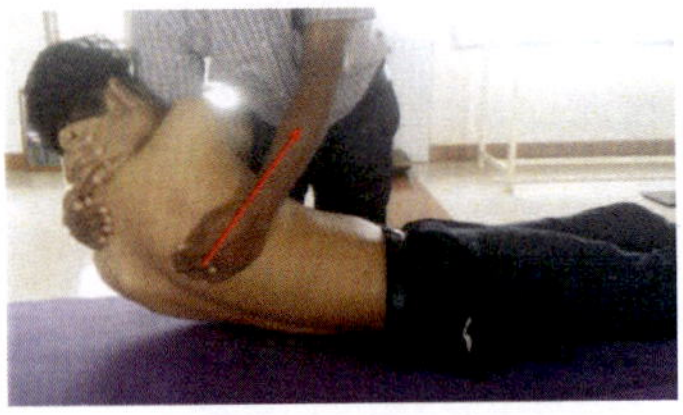
(See page no. 152)

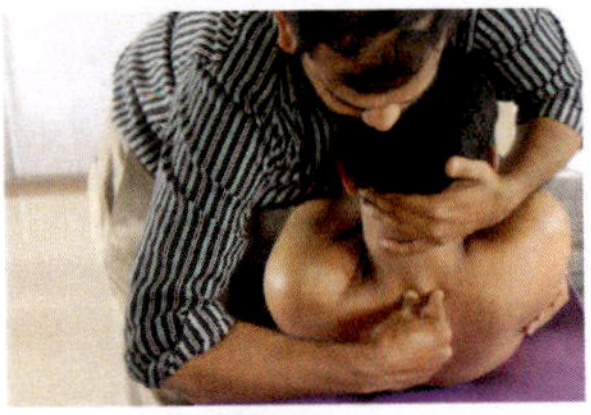
(See page no. 152)

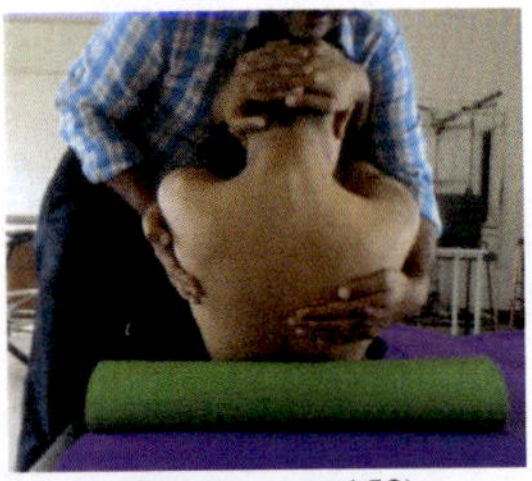
(See page no. 152)

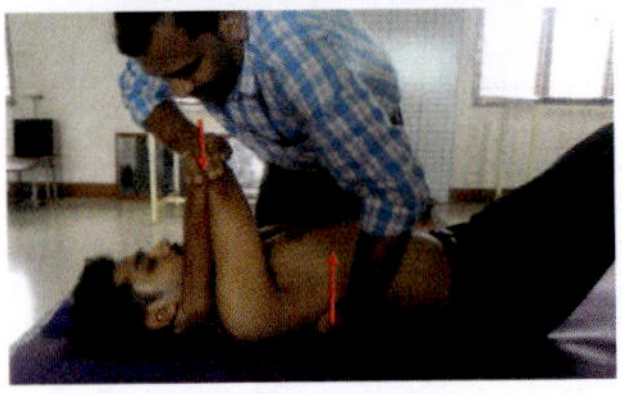
(See page no. 152)

Chapter 1

Introduction to Cardiorespiratory Physiotherapy Care

INTRODUCTION

Cardiorespiratory physiotherapy techniques can be applied to the treatment of wide range of patients with acute and chronic lung disease, but also effective in patients with advanced neuromuscular disorders, or in patients admitted to major surgeries (cardiac, thoracic and abdominal and patients on the intensive care unit. The aim is to manage breathlessness symptom control, mobility and function improvement or maintenance, and airway clearance and cough enhancement or support. Strategies and techniques include: rehabilitation, exercise testing, and exercise prescription, airway clearance, positioning and breathing techniques.

Problem List

The main problems seen with cardiorespiratory disorders are reduced lung expansion, impaired airway clearance, increased work of breathing, impaired exercise tolerance, abnormal physiologic responses to exertion, inability to meet the demands of daily living activities etc. The short term goals of rehabilitating a cardiopulmonary patient are to expand the lung which is already less aerated, to clear the secretions and to reduce the work of breathing. Long-term goals include improving exercise tolerance, patient education etc.

Techniques

Lung expansion therapy techniques are given to patients with loss of lung volume. Loss of lung volume takes a variety of forms. In atelectasis there is anatomical and physiological loss of lung volume whereas in consolidation there is only physiological loss of lung volume. Lung expansion therapy techniques are administered based on the level of consciousness. It includes positioning, breathing techniques, Neurophysiologic facilitation of respiration, mechanical aids such as CPAP and Bi PAP etc.

Secretion clearance can be a problem because of inadequate mucociliary function, impaired cough force, or excessive secretion production. Mucociliary transport can be impaired by cigarette smoking, anaesthetics, and analgesics, hypoxia or hypercapnia, dehydration, electrolyte imbalance, inhalation of dry gases, pollutants and a cuffed endotracheal tube. Cough force can be affected by pain, weakness, or incordination of the ventilator muscles. Excessive secretions are typically seen in chronic bronchitis, asthma, bronchiectasis, cystic fibrosis, and sometimes infection. So the airway clearance techniques are available to improve secretions. Bronchial hygiene therapy (Airway Clearance Techniques) involves physical or mechanical means of facilitating the removal of tracheobronchial phlegm through the external and/ or internal manipulation of airflow, and the evacuation of phlegm via coughing. So these techniques are used to mobilize and remove secretions and improve gas exchange. This includes traditional methods such as early mobilisation, positioning, and postural drainage, chest manipulations such as percussions, vibrations and shaking, breathing strategies such as active cycle breathing technique and autogenic drainage and with the help of mechanical devices such as flutter, acapella, PEP mask etc.

Work of breathing is defined as amount of pressure generated to move a certain volume of gas. Increased work of breathing in spontaneously breathing patient is manifest subjectively by breathlessness and objectively by a distressed breathing pattern. The basic principle of reducing the WOB is to optimize the balance between energy supply and demand. The basic techniques involve positioning, relaxation, breathing techniques, and the use of mechanical aids such as CPAP and BiPAP etc.

Another problem seen in cardiorespiratory patients is progressively reduced activity. A vicious cycle develops of inactivity, reduced muscular inefficiency causing increasing symptomatology and further abatement of activity in order to avoid discomfort. Exercise tolerance can be improved by aerobic conditioning. Exercise conditioning can be achieved by lower limb training, upper limb training or combined. For lower limb training walking and cycling is preferred. For combined training daily swimming or canoeing is preferred. Upper limb training is given in both obstructive disorders and restrictive disorders. For upper limb training supported exercise training is given during acute exacerbation of COPD and asthma and unsupported arm training is given during stable phase.

Another difficulty that might be encountered in patients with cardiopulmonary dysfunction is abnormal physiologic responses to increasing activity. Common abnormalities include excessive increase in heart rate, hypertensive blunted blood pressure responses, irregularities of pulses, increase in respiratory rate, oxygen desaturation etc. The appropriate therapeutic intervention for this problem is continued clinical monitoring to allow as much activity as possible while still maintaining patient safety. It is also important to instruct the patient in self monitoring of exercise intensity using pulse rate and rhythm, RPE and symptoms.

Some patients with chronic diseases become so debilitated that they are unable to meet the physical demands of the various activities of daily living they are required to perform for independence. These patients can be taught energy conservation techniques and work simplification techniques which reduces demands of the activities they must perform.

All the techniques to achieve the short-term and long-term goals are further described in succeeding chapters.

Chapter 2

Lung Expansion Therapy

INTRODUCTION

A group of techniques used to expand a collapsed lung both in conscious and unconscious patients is termed as lung expansion therapy.

Indication

Following conditions are the indications of lung expansion therapy:

- Atelectasis.
- Consolidation.
- Pleural effusion.
- Pneumothorax.
- Following abdominal surgeries and cardiac surgeries.
- Restrictive disorders of lung.

Clinical Signs of Atelectasis

- **Medical history:** Recent abdominal surgery or thoracic surgery.
- The history of chronic lung disease and cigarette consumption.
- Tachypnea and tachycardia.
- **On auscultation:** Bronchial breath sounds, fine and early inspiratory crackles may be heard.

Chest X-Ray–Signs of Atelectasis

1. Displacement of inter lobular fissure towards the affected zone.
2. Crowding of bronchopulmonary vessels in the affected region.
3. Elevation of diaphragm in the affected side.
4. Shift of trachea towards affected side.
5. Shift of mediastinum towards affected side.
6. Narrowing of space between ribs in the area of atelectasis.
7. Compensatory hyperinflation of opposite lung.
8. Shift of hilum towards the affected zone.

Mechanism of Lung Expansion Therapy

1. Increasing Transpulmonary Pressure Gradient

Transpulmonary pressure gradient is the difference between intrapulmonary pressure (IPP) and intrapleural pressure.

Intrapulmonary pressure: Air always goes from high pressure to low pressure. During inspiration the atmospheric pressure is zero and intrapulmonary pressure is negative (-1), so air goes inside. During expiration IPP is positive and atmospheric pressure is zero, so the air comes outside.

Intrapleural pressure: This pressure is negative throughout inspiration and expiration. The negativity is due two opposing forces. (1) Elastic recoil of lung tries to pull visceral pleura inwards, (2) Chest wall has a tendency to expand outwards which pulls parietal pleura outwards which is adherent to chest wall. This tendency of separation between parietal and visceral pleura creates negativity.

Any breathing techniques or a manual technique increases the negativity of Intrapleural pressure and any mechanical aids alter intrapulmonary pressure gradient. Since transpulmonary pressure gradient is the difference of these two pressures, any change in these pressures increases the transpulmonary pressure gradient thereby expanding the lungs (Figure 2.1).

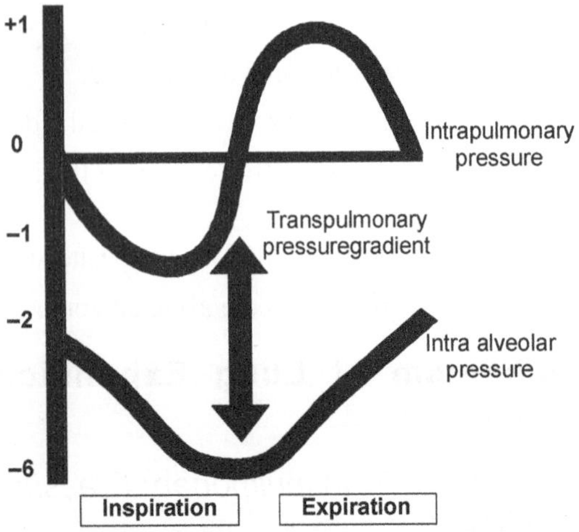

Fig. 2.1: Transpulmonary pressure gradient

2. Addition of Inspiratory Hold to Breathing Exercise will Improve Collateral Ventilation of Alveoli

Collateral channels: They are the interconnecting channels between alveoli and bronchi (Figure 2.2). They are described in Table 2.1. An addition of inspiratory hold to a breathing exercise increases this collateral ventilation thereby improving ventilation to non-aerated alveoli.

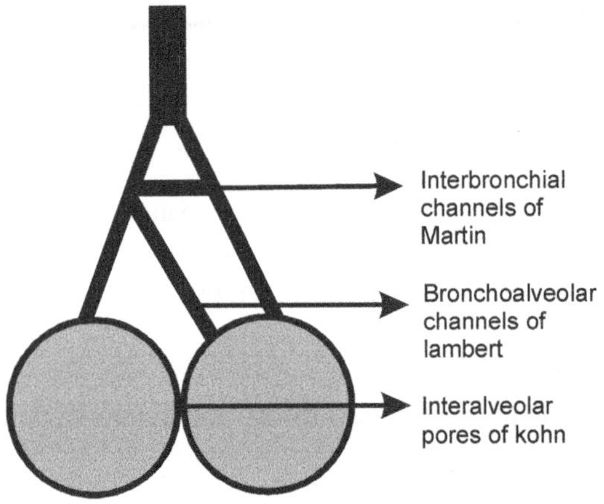

Fig. 2.2: Collateral channels

3. Physiology of Interdependence

If a group of alveoli have a tendency to collapse, the adjacent expanded alveoli produces forces that tend to prevent collapse. Since alveoli are placed closely, any techniques which expand the alveoli will also pull the non aerated alveoli from all directions. This may expand the collapsed alveoli (Figure 2.3).

Table 2.1: Types of collateral channels

Channels	*Synonym*	*Connections*
Channels of Martin	Interbronchial	Between bronchus
Channels of Lambert	Bronchoalveolar	Between bronchus and alveoli
Pores of Kohn	Interalveolar	Between alveoli

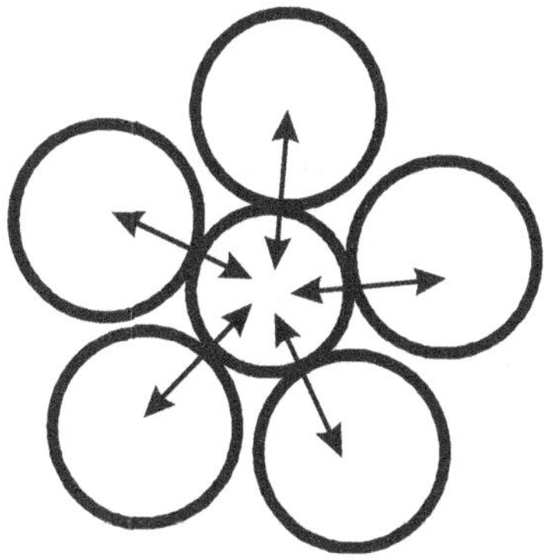

Fig. 2.3: Physiology of interdependence

(In the Figure 2.3, centre a collapsed alveoli, periphery normal aerated alveoli), each peripheral alveoli pulls the collapsed alveoli towards it (arrows).

Techniques

1. Controlled mobilization.
2. Positioning.
3. Breathing exercise.
4. Neurophysiological facilitation of respiration.
5. Incentive spirometry.
6. Intermittent positive pressure breathing (IPPB).
7. Positive pressure therapy (PEP).
8. Continuous positive airway pressure (CPAP).

Controlled Mobilization

Mobilising the patient from supine position to getting out of the bed in a slowed manner is called as controlled mobilisation. A simple walking itself increases lung volume and facilitates airway clearance in the patients. This upright posture achieved during progressive mobilisation reduces pressure on the diaphragm and encourages basal distribution of air, with natural deep breathing. (Chapter 23)

Positioning

Positioning affects the following aspects of lung function. Functional residual capacity (FRC) decreases from standing to slumped sitting. Lung compliance decreases and work of breathing increases progressively from standing, to sitting, to supine. Supine position increases shunt. Arterial oxygenation is usually higher in side lying than supine. So supine is unhelpful for lung volume. Time should be spent in side lying, well forward so that the diaphragm is free from abdominal pressure. Positioning also affects the V/Q ratio. Lying with the affected lung uppermost will make the better ventilation of the dependent normal lung is matched with better perfusion. Thus V/Q ratio is optimized and improving gas exchange. Further details are given in Chapter 5.

Breathing Exercise

Explained in Chapter 7.

Neurophysiological Facilitation of Respiration

Explained in Chapter 6.

Incentive Spirometry

Incentive spirometer decreases the intrapleural pressure thereby increasing transpulmonary pressure gradient. More explained in Chapter 8.

Intermittent Positive Pressure Breathing (IPPB)

IPPB reverses both intrapleural and intrapulmonary pressure gradient. Administration of positive pressures causes the gas to flow into the lungs. Alveolar pressures rise during the inspiratory phase of IPPB as flow occurs from the airways into the aveoli.

Positive pressure is transmitted from the aveoli to the pleural space during the inspiratory phase of an IPPB treatment, causing pleural to rise somewhat during inspiration. Depending on the mechanical properties of the lung, pleural pressure may actually exceed atmospheric pressure during a portion of inspiration. More explained in Chapter 9.

Positive Pressure Therapy (PEP)

Explained in Chapter 10.

Continuous Positive Airway Pressure (CPAP)

CPAP elevates and maintains high alveolar and airway pressures throughout the full breathing cycle. This increases transpulmonary pressure gradient throughout both inspiration and expiration. More explained in Chapter 9.

Administration of Techniques

Technique administered depends on level of consciousness:

- **If patient unconscious: PNF respiration.**
- **If patient not alert: IPPB therapy.**
- **If patient having problem with excess secretions: PEP therapy.**
- **If patient conscious and cooperative: Incentive spirometer.**
- **If problem still not resolved: Intermittent CPAP.**

Chapter 3

Bronchial Hygiene Therapy

DEFINITION

Bronchial hygiene therapy (Airway Clearance Techniques) involves the use of non-invasive airway clearance technique where physical or mechanical means of facilitating the removal of trachea-bronchial phlegm through the external and/or internal manipulation of airflow, and the evacuation of phlegm via coughing. So these techniques are used to mobilize and remove secretions and improve gas exchange.

The Normal Defence Mechanism

Particles, such as dust and soot, mold, fungi, bacteria, and viruses deposit on airway and alveolar surfaces during inhalation. Fortunately, the respiratory system has defence mechanisms to clean and protect itself. This defence mechanism is present in both upper airway and lower airway. The main defence mechanisms are sneeze reflux, cough reflux and mucociliary escalator. If the antigen passes this defence layer, specific and non-specific immunological defence mechanisms exist. The non-specific defence consists of phagocyting cells like neutrophils and macrophages and the complement activation. The specific defence mechanism (resulting in a specific immunological reaction in relation to a certain antigen) is formed by the antibodies, mainly secretary IgA and to a lesser extent IgG.

Normal Clearance

Normal airway clearance requires a patent airway, a functional mucociliary escalator, and an effective cough. Airways normally are kept open by structured support mechanisms and kept clear by proper function of their ciliated mucosa. The mucociliary clearance mechanism operates from the larynx down to the respiratory bronchioles. Ciliated epithelial cells normally move this mucus via a coordinated wave of ciliary motion toward the trachea and larynx, where excess secretions can be swallowed or expectorated.

Abnormal Clearance

Any abnormality that alters airway patency, mucociliary function, or the effectiveness of the cough reflex can impair airway clearance and cause retention of secretions.

Retention of secretions can result in full or partial airway obstruction. Full obstruction, or mucus plugging, can result in atelectasis and impaired oxygenation due to shunting. By restricting airflow, partial obstruction can increase the work of breathing and lead to air trapping, over distension, and V/Q imbalances. In the presence of pathogenic organisms, retention of secretions can lead to infection. Infectious processes, in turn, provoke an inflammatory response and the release of chemical mediators. These chemical mediators, including leukotrienes, proteases and elastases can damage the airway epithelium and increase mucus production, resulting in a vicious cycle of worsening airway clearance (Figure 3.1).

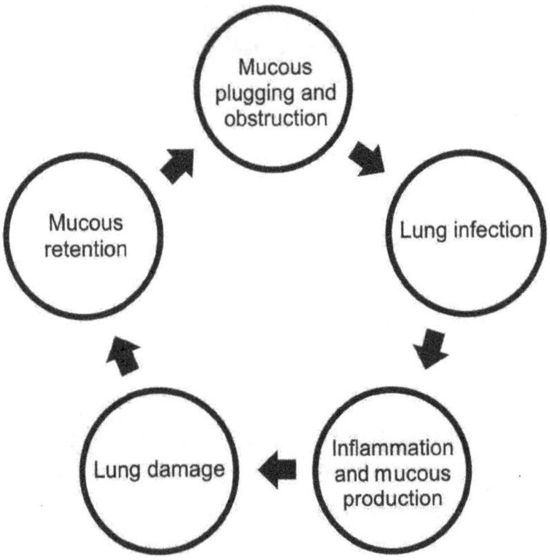

Fig. 3.1: Vicious cycle of abnormal airway clearance

Causes of Impaired Airway Clearance

Impaired airway clearance may be due to several factors which form a vicious cycle Figure 3.1. Following are the causes:

1. Mucous plugging and obstruction due to asthma.
2. Lung infection due to aspiration.
3. Inflammation and mucous production due to causes like cystic fibrosis, aspergillosis.
4. Lung damage due to abnormal gastro-oesophagial reflux.
5. Mucous retention due to causes like neuromuscular weakness, primary ciliary dyskinesia.

Indications

- **Internal obstruction or external compression:** Foreign bodies, tumors, kyphoscoliosis, bronchospasm.
- **Diseases that alter normal mucociliary clearance:** Cystic fibrosis (CF) respiratory tract cilia do not function properly, ciliary dyskinetic syndromes.
- **Chronic airway inflammation and infection:** Bronchiectasis
- **Any neurological condition that affects the four components of effective cough:** Muscular dystrophy, amyotrophic lateral sclerosis, spinal muscular atrophy, myasthenia gravis, poliomyelitis and cerebral palsy.

Determining the Need for Bronchial Hygiene Therapy

An ineffective cough, absent or increased sputum production, a labored breathing pattern, decreased breath sounds, crackles or rhonchi, tachypnea, tachycardia, or fever indicates a potential problem with retained secretions.

Interruption of Vicious Cycle

The cycle can be interrupted by following techniques:

1. Nutrition.
2. Anti-inflammatory drugs.
3. Bronchodilators.
4. Mucolytics.
5. Antibiotics.
6. Airway clearance techniques.

Various Techniques of Airway Clearance

1. Traditional Methods

a. Coughing and huffing techniques.

b. Turning.

c. Postural drainage therapy which includes:
   i. Positioning.
   ii. Postural drainage.
   iii. Percussion.
   iv. Vibration.
   v. Shaking.

d. Active mobilization.

2. Newer Methods

a. **Breathing Strategies:**
   i. Autogenic drainage.
   ii. Active cycle breathing technique (ACBT).
   iii. Forced expiratory technique (FET).

b. **Mechanical Devices:**
   i. High frequency chest wall oscillation (HFCWO).
   ii. Positive expiratory pressure therapy (PEP).
   iii. Mechanical in sufflater and ex-sufflater.
   iv. Flutter valve.
   v. Acapella.
   vi. Intrapulmonary percussive ventilator.
   vii. Cornet.
   viii. Frequencer.

ADMINISTRATION OF AIRWAY CLEARANCE TECHNIQUE BASED ON AGE

Conventional chest physiotherapy is appropriate for all age groups. For 0-1 year age group only CPT can be administered. For 1-2 years blowing games (pin wheel, bubbles) can be administered. 2-3 years HFCC can be administered. 3-4 years coughing and huffing can be administered. From four years onwards PEP, flutter or acapella can be administered. From 5 years onwards ACBT can be administered and exercise also should be encouraged as they loosen secretions. From 10 years onwards IPPV can be given. From 12 years onwards autogenic drainage can be administered.

Chapter 4

Methods to Decrease Work of Breathing

Breathlessness is defined as awareness of the intensity of breathing.
Dyspnea is difficult breathing occurring at a level of activity where it would not normally be expected.

INTRODUCTION

Work of breathing (WOB) is the work done during inspiration to overcome the resistive, elastic and inertial forces of airflow, lungs and chest wall.

DEFINITION

Work of breathing is defined as amount of pressure generated to move a certain volume of gas. It is the product of transpulmonary pressure and tidal volume. It is related to oxygen consumed by the respiratory muscles.

Facts

- WOB uses 1-4% of total body oxygen consumption at rest.
- Increased up to 40% in people with COPD.
- WOB is increased with breathlessness.

Patients are often caught in the pincer of decreased ventilator capacity and increased ventilator requirements. Increased work of breathing in spontaneously breathing patient is manifest subjectively by breathlessness and objectively by a distressed breathing pattern. The basic principle of reducing the WOB is to optimize the balance between energy supply and demand.

Measures to Optimize Balance Between Energy Supply and Demand

Measures to Increase Energy Supply

1. Nutrition management.
2. Oxygen therapy.
3. Fluid and electrolyte management.
4. Oxygen delivery to inspiratory muscles.

Measures to Decrease Energy Demand

1. Handling.
2. Sleep and rest.
3. Stress reduction.
4. Positioning.
5. Breathing re-education.
6. Mechanical assistance.
7. Exercise training.
8. Inspiratory muscle training.

Techniques

Handling Breathless People

Communication should be clear because anxiety increases oxygen consumption. Whenever interviewing a severe breathless patient questions should be such that it should have yes or no answer. Whenever the patients are getting their breath back after moving they should not be asked questions. The physical handling of acutely breathless patient requires maximum support, minimum speed and a rest between each manoeuvre.

Sleep and Rest

Fragmentation of sleep impairs respiratory performance, blunts response to hypercapnia and hypoxemia, and reduces inspiratory muscle performance. Physiotherapists should avoid waking patients unnecessarily, ensure that their treatment does not cause fatigue and contribute to the teamwork required to allow adequate sleep.

Positioning

A COPD patient assumes a posture with a poked chin (flexion of lower cervical column with hyperextension of upper cervical column. The arms are outreached and supported on the chair or table. When the distal part of upper limb is fixed (arms in supported position) the ribcage can move on shoulder and take part in respiration. This can optimize accessory muscle function. If a towel roll is placed under the lumbar vertebrae, this can result in lordosis and anterior pelvic tilt position. This also enhances the accessory muscle function. Also there are positions which optimize the length tension status of the diaphragm.

The different positions used to relieve breathlessness are:

- Forward lean sitting.
- Forward lean standing.
- Relaxed sitting.
- Relaxed standing.
- Side lying.
- High side lying.
- Breathless children may prefer a kneeling position.

In first and second positions, the abdominal contents raise the anterior part of the diaphragm, possibly facilitating its contraction during inspiration. A similar effect can be seen in the side lying and high side lying positions where the curvature of the dependent part of the diaphragm is increased. This effect combined with relaxation of the head, neck and shoulders promotes the pattern of breathing control.

Relaxation

Patients should be warm, comfortable and have adequate fresh air. Deeper relaxation may be achieved by learning a relaxation technique like Jacobson relaxation or Mitchell relaxation.

Breathing Techniques used in Reducing Work of Breathing

1. Breathing control technique.
2. Innocenti technique.
3. Pursed lip breathing.

Explained in Chapter 7.

Tips to Reduce Breathlessness

- **Avoidance of breath holding:** Breath holding increases tension and breathlessness. Breath holding can be observed when patients are concentrating, making an effort or listening to advice. Whenever physiotherapist or family members are first to notice this, it is better to advice them so they can control their breathlessness.

- A fan reduces the breathlessness by influencing the receptors in the trigeminal nerve distribution that provides information to sensory cortex.
- Studies have shown that mechanical vibration over chest wall can reduce breathlessness.
- Self acupressure to any of the following breathless points:
  - Anterior midline between nipples at the level of 4th intercostal space.
  - Just below each coracoid process.
  - One and half thumb width lateral to lower border of each T3 spinous process.

Mechanical Aids to Deliver Non-Invasive Ventilation

Non-invasive ventilation provides inspiratory muscle rest for people who are burdened with ventilator failure due to excessive work of breathing. It unloads inspiratory muscles, reduces breathlessness and corrects respiratory acidosis. The common modes used are CPAP, IPPB and BiPAP.

Chapter 5

Therapeutic Body Positioning

DEFINITION

Therapeutic Body Positioning can be defined as primary non-invasive physical therapy intervention that can augment arterial oxygenation. So that invasive, mechanical, pharmacological forms of respiratory support can be postponed or reduced or avoided.

Routine body positioning, is done by nurses. Mechanical body positioning also called as kinetic therapy is performed to prevent respiratory complications such as Ventilator associated pneumonia.

USES OF BODY POSITIONING

1. Minimize the work of breathing, i.e., promote efficient diaphragm and accessory muscle function.
2. Promote airway clearance.
3. Improved expansion of targeted region of the lungs based on specific positioning of that region.
4. Optimize relaxation.
5. Provide pain relief.
6. Improve ventilation, ventilation-perfusion matching and gas exchange.
7. Minimize dyspnea.

AIMS

Respiratory System

- Mechanics
  - Alters chest wall configuration.
  - Improves lung volume and capacities.
  - To maintain optimal position of the diaphragm.
  - Enhances abdominothoracic breathing.
- To improve expansion of lungs
  - Improves regional ventilation, perfusion and diffusion.
  - Improves V/Q matching.
- To improve secretion clearance
  - Improves mucociliary transport.
  - Stimulate effective and productive cough.
- To reduce work of breathing
  - Improves respiratory muscle efficacy.
  - Reduces airway resistance.
  - Promote relaxation.

Cardiovascular System

- Enhanced venous and lymphatic drainage.
- Prevents gravitational, mechanical and compression forces on the myocardium, mediastinal structures and great vessels.

- Fluid shift from central to dependent areas if needed.
- Minimises orthostatic hypotension.

Central Nervous System

- Increases patients arousal.
- Reduces intracranial pressure.
- Alters muscle tone.
- Alters abnormal postural tone.

Others

- Prevents skin breakdown.
- Prevents contractures.
- Increases chest tube drainage.
- Increases urinary drainage.

All positions used as cardiorespiratory techniques is discussed below in terms of Pulmonary mechanics, Cardiovascular mechanics, Ventilation, Perfusion, V/Q matching, Beneficial and hazardous effects.

UPRIGHT POSITION

Uses

- All movements to upper limbs are given in this position.
- Upright position with legs dependent is the standard reference position for pulmonary function testing.
- Forced expiratory maneuvers including coughing should be encouraged in upright position.

Pulmonary Mechanics

Rib cage assumes greater anteroposterior diameter. Compression on heart and lungs is minimal, so the vertical gravitational gradient is maximal. All lung volume and capacities increases in this position except closing volume. FRC is greater in standing then in sitting than in supine position. Higher the FRC less the airway closure more the arterial oxygenation. Diameter of main airway is increased which results in reduction of airway resistance. Since abdomen is away from diaphragm, these fibres are in shortened position. This result in reduction of muscle force generated. Tonic abdominal activity is a counteracting mechanism for this shortened position. This increases the muscle efficacy.

Cardiovascular Mechanics

There will be redistribution of venous volume with secondary changes in ventricular filling and cardiac output. CV System has to work harder to maintain its cardiac output due to decrease in venous return. A 90 mm of driving force of calf muscles is required to prevent back flow of blood between contractions. Muscles work in combination with valves. Respiratory system acts as pump during inspiration where intrathoracic pressure becomes more negative. This result in reduced Right atrial pressure, reduced SV and increased heart rate.

Distribution of Ventilation

The pleural pressure is less negative from the apex to the base of the lungs. So in the apex these lung units have larger initial lung volume, hence small volume changes occur with inspiration. The lung units at the base have smaller initial lung volume thus larger volume changes occur during respiration. Breathing at low lung volume reverses the normal intra pleural pressure gradient. Compare with bases which have a positive intrapleural pressure that exceeds airway pressure apex is better ventilated than bases. So the bases are prone to airway closure in individuals breathing at low lung volume. Breathing at mechanical ventilation again reverses the intrapleural pressure and apex is better ventilated. Whenever pleural pressure is greater than airway pressures, airways are closed and the region is not ventilated.

Distribution of Perfusion

Distribution of perfusion is also dependent on gravity. For further explanations; please note the abbreviations of the variables: Alveolar pressure is denoted as P_A, Pulmonary arterial pressure is denoted as P_a and venous pressure is denoted as P_V.

Lung perfusion is divided into four zones where zone I is uppermost and zone IV is lowermost.

Zone I: $P_A > P_a > P_V$

As alveolar pressure is higher than arterial pressure in zone I, the blood vessels are closed. However under normal conditions, the P_a is sufficient to maintain some flow which predominates in the corner vessels.

Zone II: $P_a > P_A > P_V$

In zone II arterial pressure is higher than alveolar pressure. Here the blood flow is pulsatile with reduced volume during diastole. The middle zone or zone II reflects the blood flow from the recruitment of blood vessels.

Zone III: $P_a > P_V > P_A$

Here both arterial and venous pressure is more than alveolar pressure. The flow is more, sustained and majority of vessels are patent. Zone III reflects the blood flow from the distension of pulmonary vessels.

Zone IV

Zone IV refers to the base of the lungs. Here there is no flow. This is because interstitial pressure acting on the pulmonary blood vessels and creating a compression force. And also because of weight of the lungs can also account for minimal flow.

A decrease arterial pressure due to RHF or decreased circulating volume results in development of zone I in lung. Increased arterial pressure during exercise or left to right intra cardiac shunt results in recruitment of upper lungs. The presence of obstructive lung disease or positive pressure ventilation increases P_A disproportional to P_a, so that the presence of zone I in lung become significant and physiologic dead space also increases.

V/Q Matching

Both ventilation and perfusion increases from apex to base of upright lung. Perfusion increases greater extent than ventilation so that V/Q ratio decreases from apex to base. As a result V/Q ratio is high at apex and low at base. It approaches 0.8 in zone II of the lungs.

Tissue Oxygenation

Mascular and cutaneous vasoconstriction occur to ensure blood flow is maintained to vital organ such as heart and brain. Diffusion region below the level of heart have greater driving pressure which promotes diffusion than those above heart.

SUPINE POSITIONING

Uses

- Commonly used position for surgical and other invasive procedures.
- It serves as reference position for hemo-dynamic measures.
- Common position used for basic care.
- Most prolonged position used for critically ill patients.

Pulmonary Mechanics

AP diameter of abdomen and rib cage decreased and increased laterally. Hemidiaphragm is displaced upwards (towards head) due to increased abdominal pressure. Thus FRC can be reduced due to shift of diaphragm and increased thoracic blood volume. Since FRC is reduced and CV remains same, there will be early airway closure. Excess secretions tend to pool in dependent side of airway. There will be reduction in lung compliance both (static, dynamic) in supine positioning, as a result of increased pulmonary blood volume and airway closure. There will be increased airway resistance in supine due to reduced FRC. All these effects pre dispose the patient to airway closure and increase WOB (because closing volume remain similar to that in sitting and thus exceed FRC.

Cephalad shift of diaphragm places it at a mechanical advantage so that tidal volume is predominately generated by diaphragm abdominal displacement. Thus, the mechanical load to breath that is the driving pressure increases to maintain minute ventilation.

Cardiovascular Mechanics

There will be central shift of blood volume from extremities to central circulation which initiates orthostatic hypotension. This fluid shift increases both preload and after load of right side of heart. This increased volume tends to distort the interventricular septum and reduces left ventricular volume and its pre load.

Distribution of Ventilation

There will be 30% reduction in vertical height of the lung which results in small intrapleural pressure gradient which suggest that distribution of ventilation would be more uniform than upright lung. In subject with significant airway closure, however the gradient becomes more uniform since the dependent airways are closed at onset of inspiration. This is due to large dependent lung surface area and decrease in FRC. Cephalad zones are better ventilated than caudal or diaphragmatic zones because of weight of caudal mediastinum, abdominal hydrostatic pressure and distortion of dependent ribcage.

Distribution of Perfusion

The distribution of perfusion is more uniform throughout the lung. Since P_a and P_V exceed P_A, entire lung is predominated by zone III. In subjects with airway closure, perfusion is greater to non-dependent lung due to hypoxic vasoconstriction further due to dependent airway closure prevalent in supine position.

V/Q Ratio

V/Q ratio increases from the non-dependent to dependent lung region. This is primarily due to change in ventilation. This regional difference in V/Q ratio is smaller compared to upright positioning.

Beneficial Effect of Supine

- Better V/Q matching.
- Less resting length of diaphragm.

Hazardous Effects of Supine

- Reduced FRC.
- Reduced vital capacity.
- Reduced flow rates.
- Increased area of dependent lung.
- Increased closure of dependent airways.

SIDE LYING POSITION

Uses

- Most common position used for unilateral lung pathologies.
- For acidity and Gastro-oesophagial disease, subjects lies on left side.

Pulmonary Mechanics

In side lying at rest AP diameter increased and lateral diameter decreased. There is an increase in lateral excursion of rib cage of non-dependent zone. The anteroposterior excursions of rib cage increase or decrease while those of abdomen decrease. Thus diameters and tidal excursions change in opposite directions. This mechanism is due to difference in distribution of respiratory muscle force, activity or mechanical advantage of various inspiratory muscles and local compliance in rib cage and abdomen. The FRC in side lying is intermittent between upright and supine. The regional FRC is greater in non-dependent lung. There will be increased WOB in side lying compared to upright due to decreased compliance, increased resistance and abdominal pressure.

Minute ventilation is lower than that in sitting on side lying due to fewer fibers are stretched by cephalic displacement in dependent zone. AP displacement of abdomen in side lying position may decrease the base on which diaphragm acts to expand the rib cage thus decreasing its efficacy.

Cardiovascular Mechanics

Left ventricular end diastolic pressure increased in left side lying due to position induced reduction in left ventricular compliance. Right ventricular precordium, extra cardiac intrathoracic structures and higher intra-abdominal organ could act to compress left ventricle.

Ventilation

Initial ventilation gradient decreases from upper to lower lung and vertical ventilation gradient increases from upper to lower lungs. Cephalocaudal gradient is intermediate in magnitude between supine and prone positioning predominates in dependent lung.

Perfusion

Perfusion increases from non-dependent to dependent region of lungs at a greater magnitude than in supine or prone positioning. Upper one third of each lung is in zone II, while lower two third is in zone III.

V/Q Ratio

It is lowest at point 20 cm from dependent aspect of lower lung and increased both above below this point, regardless of whether subject was in left or right side lying position. There is overall decrease in V/Q ratio from non-dependent region of upper lung to dependent region of lower lung.

- Optimal V/Q matching occurs upper 1/3rd of each lung.
- For bilateral lung pathology make the patient lie on right side.
- In left side lying, there will be compression of heart over lungs.

PRONE POSITIONING

Types

The two common variants of the prone position are Prone abdomen restricted and Prone abdomen free position. Prone abdomen restricted refers to lying prone with the abdomen in contact with the bed, whereas in the prone abdomen free position, the patient's hips and chest are elevated so that the abdomen is free.

Uses

- This position improves oxygenation and reduces work of breathing in patients with cardiopulmonary dysfunction.
- The most common position used for ARDS patients.

Pulmonary Mechanics

In this position diameter is same as supine even though AP diameter decreased in abdomen. There will be more decrease in abdominal AP excursion but the excursion remains greater than that of then lateral excursion. Diaphragm is displaced by abdominal contents which enhances its mechanical advantage so that it can oppose increased abdominal pressure. FRC is greater than supine but less than sitting. FRC of prone abdominal free position is greater than prone abdominal restricted position. Lung compliance is decreased than supine due to decreased compliance of the rib cage and diaphragm.

Cardiovascular Mechanics

There will be more compression of the heart due to location of heavy mass above the heart. The fluid shift from limbs to thorax is same as that of supine.

Ventilation

Lung undergoes decrease in vertical height. Expansion gradient is less than that of upright lungs in both prone positions. In typical prone position ventilation is distributed uniformly in the vertical direction. In prone abdomen free position ventilation is greater in dependent zones. There is greater caudal ventilation in prone position and greater cephalad ventilation in prone abdomen free position.

V/Q Ratio

Ratio is same as that of supine.

Beneficial Effects

- It increases oxygenation, tidal volume, dynamic compliance.
- Uniform V/Q matching.
- Uniform pleural pressure gradient due to less compression of lungs by heart.
- Reduces stroke volume and increases sympathetic activity.
- It augments urine output.

Hazardous Effects

- Skin breakdown
- Pressure points stress on head and face.
- Stress on tubing and circuitry of mechanical ventilation.
- Alveoli in the base one compressed by weight of lungs, heavy with blood, pressure from abdominal content once the potential to expand.

Note:

Effect of body position on bronchiolar diameter

When upright, the diameter of main airway increases. If the airways are obstructed even small degrees of airway narrowing induced by recumbency can result in significant airway resistance.

Effect of body position on drainage from pelvis of the kidney

Promotion of urinary drainage from renal pelvis to the bladder when in upright position, as a result of reduced area for urinary stasis when in this position as opposed to the supine position.

Effect of body position on distribution of mucus within bronchi

Excess secretion tends to pool on dependent side of airway.

Non-dependent side may dry out exposing the patient to infection and obstruction.

POSITIONING IN RESTRICTIVE DISORDERS

Positioning in Pleural Effusion

People with moderate pleural effusion may benefit from side lying with affected side uppermost because ventilation and perfusion are greater in lower lung, there will be optimal V/Q matching. Larger effusions are more likely to show improvement of oxygenation with affected side lowermost because this can minimise compression of unaffected lung.

Positioning in Pneumothorax

Lying on good side is often most comfortable and there will be optimal V/Q matching. Lying on affected side may speed the absorption of the air.

Positioning in Bronchiectasis

In case of unilateral bronchiectasis leg end is often elevated even in the night with effected side uppermost. This will optimize V/Q ratio and better drainage of secretions. In case of bilateral bronchiectasis patient should lie on supine position with leg end elevation. A leg end elevation can be achieved by keeping bricks under the couch.

Positioning in Unilateral Lung Pathology

Unilateral lung pathologies like atelectasis, consolidation, effusions and operated conditions like lobectomy the affected side or the operated side should be uppermost (bad lung up rule). Ventilation and perfusion are usually matched because the better-ventilated dependent lung is also better perfused. For people with one-sided pneumonia, reduced ventilation on the affected side overrides the physiological ventilation gradient. When the patient lies with the affected lung uppermost, the better ventilation of the dependent normal lung is matched with better perfusion. Perfusion is always greater in dependent areas, and V_A/Q match is therefore enhanced in the 'bad lung up' position, sometimes resulting in a dramatic improvement in gas exchange. V_A/Q is usually mismatched if the affected lung is dependent.

As well as optimizing gas exchange, 'bad lung up rule' suits other situations. It promotes comfort following thoracotomy or chest drain placement, facilitates postural drainage, and help in improving lung volume when atelectatic lung is positioned uppermost to encourage expansion. With atelectasis, the uppermost areas are stretched and better expanded, even though the dependent lung may be better ventilated because of the compressed alveoli having greater potential to expand and take in fresh gas.

Exceptions to Bad Lung Up Rule

- **Recent pneumonectomy:** When patient lie on operated side, fibrin and fluid deposition takes place in the empty thorax. Hence mediastinal herniation to operated side can be minimized.
- **Large pleural effusion:** Mechanism explained above.
- **Bronchopleural fistula:** In this case any unwanted substances drain into the unaffected dependent lung.
- **A large main stem bronchus tumour:** If patient is positioned with operated side uppermost may obstruct the bronchus and cause breathlessness.
- Whenever patients show discomfort.
- Sudden reduction in saturation.

POSITIONING IN OBSTRUCTIVE DISORDERS

During acute exacerbation of asthma or COPD, the patient's accessory muscles should be facilitated. An anterior pelvic tilt facilitates accessory muscle use. This can be achieved by placing a towel roll vertically along the spine in supine. During the stable phase the pelvis should be posteriorly tilted to facilitate diaphragmatic muscle. This can be achieved by placing a pillow under the knees. There are some other positions used during breathlessness episodes during ADL's. These positions and its rationale are described below.

The patient can put into any of the following positions and encouraged to do diaphragmatic breathing (breathing control) at his own rate. Once the patient gains control of breathing, he should be encouraged to slow down his respiratory rate. Patients with a flat diaphragm may benefit from some of the positions that use pressure from abdominal contents to dome the muscle and provide some stretch to its fibers so that it can work with greater efficiency. The arms are best supported, to optimize accessory muscle functions. In these positions, the serratus anterior, latissmus dorsi and pectoral muscle are used in their reversed action to assist in thoracic expansion.

Following are the positions used for recovery from shortness of breath:

1. High Side Lying

Five or six pillows are used to raise the patient's shoulders while lying on his side. One pillow should be placed between the waist and axilla, to keep the spine straight and prevent slipping down the bed. The top pillow must be above the shoulders, so that only the head and neck are supported. The underneath forearm can be placed under the head pillow, or resting on the bed underneath the pillow in the waist. It is more comfortable if the knees are bent and the top leg placed in front of the one beneath. This position is helpful for patients in respiratory distress or those who suffer from acute breathless or orthopnea during the night.

2. Forward Lean Sitting

The patients sit at the table leaning forward from the hips with head and upper chest supported on several (two to three) pillows. The back must be kept straight, so that diaphragmatic movement is not inhibited. Care should be taken that the patient maintains a straight thoracic and lumbar spine as otherwise tend to inhibit diaphragmatic movement.

3. Kneeling (Especially for Children)

Children can sit or kneel with the head and upper chest resting against pillows.

4. Relaxed Sitting

The patient should sit upright in a chair with supported arms. This is the easiest position that can be taken up easily. The back should be kept straight, with the forearms resting on the thighs and the wrists relaxed.

5. Forward Lean Standing

If they are unable to sit down, distressed patients are inclined to grasp the nearest available object and hold themselves in a tense position; for insurance they hold on to the banisters after climbing a flight of stairs. They should be encouraged to lean forward with the forearms resting on an object of suitable height such as windowsill or banisters.

6. Relaxed Standing

The patient can lean back against a wall with the feet placed slightly apart and approximately 30 cm away from it. The shoulders and arms should be relaxed and hanging loosely by sides.

7. Stride Standing

Standing relaxed leaning sideways against a wall, arms in pockets, if support is needed for the accessory muscles.

8. Occasional Positions

a. Lying flat as this put pressure from the abdominal contents against the diaphragm.

b. A few patients even find a slight head down tilt is also helpful.

Chapter 6

Neurophysiological Facilitation of Respiration

HISTORY

Bethune 1975, Ontario, Canada.

DEFINITION

Externally applied proprioceptive and tactile stimuli that produce reflex respiratory movement response and that appear to alter the rate and depth of breathing.

RATIONALE

- Monotonous or shallow respiration leads to inadequate ventilation which leads to atelectasis and retention of secretions.
- Lack of muscle tone leads to instability of chest wall which, further leads to deranged mechanical respiratory dysfunction.

TECHNIQUES

1. Perioral pressure.
2. Intercostal stretch.
3. Manual vertebral pressure (High).
4. Manual vertebral pressure (Low).
5. Co-contraction of abdomen.
6. Anterior stretch basal lift.
7. Maintained moderate manual pressure.

Each technique discussed under stimulus, response and suggested mechanism.

1. Perioral Pressure

Stimulus: Applying firm maintained pressure to the patients on upper lip.

Response: Five seconds apnea followed by epigastric excursion, deep breathing, and mouth closure and swallowing altogether called as snout phenomena.

Suggested mechanism: Primitive reflex response related to sucking breathing and swallowing.

2. Intercostal Stretch

Stimulus: Applying pressure to upper border of lower rib in order to stretch the intercostals muscle in downward direction.

Response: Gradual increase in respiratory movements in area under and around stretch.

Suggested mechanism: Through intercostal stretch receptors.

3. Manual Vertebral Pressure (High)

Stimulus: Manual pressure to thoracic vertebral region of T2 – T5.

Response: Increased epigastric excursion and deep breathing.

Suggested mechanism: Through dorsal root mediated inter-segmental reflex.

4. Manual Vertebral Pressure (Low)

Stimulus: Manual pressure to thoracic vertebral region of T7–T10.

Response: Increased respiratory movements of apical thorax.

Suggested mechanism: Dorsal root mediated inter-segmental reflex.

5. Co-contraction of Abdomen

Stimulus: Therapist placing one hand on patients' lower ribs and one pelvis on same side and pushing with moderate pressure so that force is applied right angle to the patient.

Response: Increased epigastric excursion, increased muscle contraction of rectus abdominis, decrease girth in obese, increase firmness to palpation and coughing.

Suggested mechanism: Through stretch receptors of abdominal muscles and inter-costal to phrenic reflexes.

6. Anterior Stretch Basal Lift

Stimulus: Procedure is performed by placing hands under posterior ribs of supine patient and lifting gently upwards.

Response: Increased expansion of posterior basal area.

Suggested mechanism: Through dorsal root mediated inter-segmental reflex stretch receptors in intercostals and back muscles.

7. Maintained Moderate Manual Pressure

Stimulus: Mild pressure of open hands is maintained over the area in which expansion is desired.

Response: Gradually increased excursion on area of contact.

Suggested mechanism: Cutaneous afferent.

GENERAL EFFECTS OF ALL THE PROCEDURES

- Changes in breath sound as determined by auscultation have been noted with all procedures.
- Some unconscious patients appear to become less deeply unconscious during respiratory facilitation.
- Response such as fluttering eye lids, head movements, spontaneous movements, opening of eyes.

Factors that Alter Response

- Patients' pre-existing muscle tone.
- Level of consciousness.
- Adequacy of ventilation.
- Obesity.

Contraindications

- Abdominal co-contractions is avoided in patients with decerebrate rigidity, young children.
- Inter-costal stretch in fractured rib.
- In children except peri-oral stimulation all other procedures are contraindicated.

Chapter 7

Breathing Techniques/Exercises

INTRODUCTION

Reduced lung expansion, accumulation of secretions and increased work of breathing are main problems seen with respiratory disorders. Physiotherapists use Lung expansion therapy, Bronchial hygiene therapy and PT techniques to reduce work of breathing to address the above problems. Breathing exercises is an important component in all of the above techniques. Breathing techniques can be divided into normal breathing, known as 'breathing control', where minimal effort is expended, and breathing exercises where either inspiration is emphasized as in thoracic expansion exercises or expiration is emphasized as in the huff of the forced expiration technique.

DEFINITION

Breathing exercise can be defined as the therapeutic intervention by which purpose full alteration of a given breathing pattern are categorized as breathing exercises. Outcomes have ranged from to increase lung volume, to clear secretions, to improve gas exchange, to control breathlessness, to increase exercise capacity, to reduce blood pressure, to reduce obesity, relaxation response for stress reduction and to control pain in natural child birth.

CLASSIFICATION

Breathing exercise can be classified as inspiratory and expiratory. Some of the breathing exercises stresses inspiration thereby increasing lung volume whereas others stresses on expiration which assists in clearance of secretions.

Breathing Techniques in Respiratory Disorders

In restrictive types of disorders Deep Breathing, Diaphragmatic Breathing, Deep Diaphragmatic Breathing, End-Inspiratory hold, Sustained Maximal Inspiration, Slow Maximal Inspiration, Incentive Spirometer, Sniff, Segmental (Apical and Lateral Costal Activity) are commonly used. Abdominal Breathing, Air Shift Breathing, Glossopharyngeal Breathing are commonly effective in spinal cord injuries. Stacked Breathing, Air Shift Breathing are used in localized and generalised atelectasis of upper lobe respectively. Chest mobility exercises and Belt exercises are used to prevent the formation of disabling adhesions between two layers of pleura.

1. In deep breathing subjects were asked to breathe in deeply and slowly through the nose and sigh out through the mouth. Breathing through nose warms and humidifies air but doubles resistance to air flow. Inspiration is slow to decrease velocity and increase the

strength of muscle contraction. Expiration is through the mouth to keep the airway open patency of small airway closure.

2. In diaphragmatic breathing, the subjects were asked to get comfortable position. They were instructed to rest the dominant hand on their abdomen with elbows supported and keeping their shoulder relaxed. Allow their hand to rise gently while visualizing air filling the abdomen like a balloon. Progress this exercises to side lying and relaxed standing.
3. Deep diaphragmatic breathing is a combination of deep breathing with diaphragmatic breathing.
4. End-inspiratory technique can be administered along with deep diaphragmatic breathing to further stress the inspiration. When there is a region of lung which has partial obstructed airway or decreased compliance, the alveoli will fill at a slower rate than the unaffected areas that is increased time constant. Patients with airway disease or scattered areas of atelectasis have local variations of time constants. These areas need more time to expand than unaffected areas, therefore slow deep breathing with a hold on inspiration allows them more chance of gaining ventilation. Holding the breath allows time for the air to diffuse through collateral channels. It is not suitable for breathless people.
5. Sniff is a simple and effective technique used to increase diaphragmatic excursion further along with deep diaphragmatic exercises. It augments collateral circulation. Perform the normal diaphragmatic breathing exercise as mentioned above. Then ask the subject to sniff in three times. During exhalation, tell the subjects to let it out slow which help to decrease RR and some relaxation. Progressively decrease the no. of sniffs as the day progresses.
6. Segmental exercise: Hypoventilation does occur in certain areas of the lungs because of chest wall fibrosis, pain, and muscle guarding after surgery, atelectasis and pneumonia. So in these circumstances Segmental exercises can be given to increase localised expansion of the lungs. The techniques used with segmental exercises may elicit localised drop in intrapleural pressure thereby increasing transpulmonary pressure gradient which results in expansion. Manual cues such as vibration or pressure sensation are provided over the regions of chest wall that is not expanding well may also aid in expansion. It is preferable to teach unilateral basal expansion exercises otherwise the patient is unable to relax the shoulder girdle adequately and this tends to exaggerate the movement of the upper chest. Three types of segmental breathing that target the apical, lateral and posterior segments of the lower lobes are apical expansion exercises, lateral costal breathing and posterior basal expansion exercises. They should not be performed during attacks of breathless.
7. The following technique further stresses inspiration. First squeeze chest during expiration then stretch at the very end of expiration, allow inspiration to occur. Near the end of inspiration apply a series of 3 or 4 gentle stretches rather similar to repeated contractions.
8. Stacked breathing is the only breathing exercise where there is more inspiratory efforts given compared to a single expiratory effort. In this technique subjects have to breathe in 3-4 times without expiration, each time filling the lung a little bit more up to vital capacity. This exercise is better fit for individuals with weak respiratory muscles to achieve full inspiration prior to a cough. A glottis closure between each attempt allows a buildup of extra volume within the lungs, thereby achieving a good laryngeal control. This technique is used to enhance the stage 2 of coughing technique training. Stacked breathing technique is also used mainly for unilateral localised collapses.

9. In a slow maximal inspiration, subject asked to do slow inspiration for as long as possible. This keeps the glottis open and air can continue to move. This encourages recruitment of all muscle fibers.

10. A sustained maximal inspiration is a slow, deep inhalation from FRC up to the total lung capacity, followed by 5 to 10 sec breath hold. An SMI is thus functionally equivalent to performing an inspiratory capacity maneuver, followed by a breath hold. In slow maximal inspiration, patient sustains to act of slow inspiration for as long as possible. This keeps the glottis open and air can continue to move. This encourage recruitment of all muscle fibers. Both of these techniques can increase lung expansion by altering transpulmonary pressure gradient, boosting collateral ventilation and improving the physiology of interdependence. Incentive Spirometry which was developed by Barlett *et al.* uses the principle of sustained maximal inspiration. It was designed to mimic natural sighing or yawning by encouraging the subject to take long slow deep breaths and hold.

11. Glossopharyngeal breathing is indicated in subjects with severe weakness of muscles of inspiration like high spinal cord injury. This technique is often called frog breathing and involves using the tongue to move air into the lungs. Procedure is such that subject takes several gulps of air. Then the mouth is closed, tongue pushes the air back and traps it in the pharynx, air is then forced into the lungs when glottis is opened. Each gulp of air delivers 60 to 200 mL of air to the inspiratory volume. Six to nine gulps are stacked together for its effectiveness. This technique increases the depth of inspiration, vital capacity, peak expiratory flow rate and maximal voluntary ventilation.

12. Abdominal breathing exercise is the only breathing exercise where expiration is done first followed by inspiration. This exercise is indicated in subjects who are paralysed or extremely weak diaphragms but with good abdominal and accessory muscle strength. The procedure includes contraction of abdominal muscles tightly followed by its relaxation. Muscle contraction increases abdominal pressure pushes the diaphragm to unusually high position in thorax. When abdominal muscles are relaxed the diaphragm passively falls to produce expiration accessory muscles can assist with this inspiratory effort to produce greater tidal volume. The disadvantages are every time to breathe in a conscious effort is necessary, subject must be in upright position to provide this exercise and subjects require mechanical ventilation during lying and sleep.

13. Airshift breathing: Any individual with paradoxical breathing or a poorly expanding chest wall during inspiration should learn to perform an airshift maneuver. When an individual has a dominant diaphragmatic breathing pattern that results in collapse of the anterior chest wall (as occurs in those with C4-T4 motor complete injuries), the volume of air moving into lungs does not act to expand the chest wall but instead moves in a caudal direction. An air shift is a maneuver in which a person inhales maximally, closes the glottis and relaxes the diaphragm to the individual to move the air upward toward the middle and upper lobes of the chest and creates expansion of these regions. It can potentially expand the chest from half to 2 inch. Position the patient in supine lying. Practice with opening mouth. Ask the patient to take deep breath and hold that breath. While holding the breath, therapist asks the patient to tuck in the abdomen so that air will move from lower part to upper part of thorax. Instruct the patient to perform this exercise daily. With Airshift technique,

chest mobility can be maintained for subjects who are with good chest wall range of motion and intercostals muscle weakness. The uses are to increase ROM of chest and a method of learning laryngeal control. As both Airshift and stacked breathing techniques used for achieving laryngeal control, they can be used for better effectiveness (stage 2) of cough. Airshift Maneuver can be used also for generalized collapses. The possible complications arc consequences associated with breath holding and hyperventilation. To avoid this, individual should exhale between attempts and should rest frequently in the training sessions.

Chest mobility exercises and Belt exercises are used to prevent the formation of disabling adhesions between two layers of pleura.

14. Chest mobilization exercises can be defined as any exercises that combine active movements of the trunk or extremities with deep breathing. They are designed to maintain or improve mobility of the chest wall, trunk, and shoulder girdles when it affects ventilation or postural alignment. These exercises are indicated mainly in pleural disorders, especially after ICD removal for increasing mobility of one side of thorax and preventing adhesions between two layers of pleura. Further details are explained in Chapter 25.

15. Belt exercises serve the purpose same as that of chest mobility exercise where the difference is that reinforcement over the chest is given with the help of a rolled bed sheet or a belt. Belt exercises aid in increasing the mobility of lateral basal (unilateral and bilateral) and posterior basal segments.

    Impaired airway clearance can be interrupted by mucolytics, nutrition, bronchodilators, anti-inflammatories, antibiotics and airway clearance techniques. Airway clearance techniques or bronchohygiene therapy includes traditional methods like coughing, huffing and manual drainage techniques such as postural drainage, percussion, vibration and shaking whereas newer methods includes mechanical devices like high frequency oscillation, positive expiratory pressure mask, flutter valve, intrapulmonary percussive ventilator and breathing strategies such as autogenic drainage (AD) and active cycle breathing technique (ACBT). They foster independence because once taught they can be used without assistance. They are suited for the people with chronic lung problems.

16. ACBT consists of three phases breathing control, thoracic expansion and forced expiratory technique (FET). FET consists of low huffs and high huffs interspersed with breathing control. Details are given in Chapter 16.

17. AD is a method of controlled breathing in which patient adjust the rate, location and depth of respiration. It can be of Belgian approach and German approach. Belgian approach is divided into three phases such as unsticky phase, collecting phase and evacuating phase whereas German approach has only one phase. Details are given in Chapter 15.

    In patients with obstructive disorders there will be reduction of flow rate and increase in residual volume and total lung capacities. They predominantly use accessory muscles so work of breathing is increased. So goals of the management are to change the breathing pattern, reduce work of breathing and use more of energy conservation techniques. These types of patients have a period of acute exacerbation followed by their stable phase. Breathing Control Technique, Innocenti Technique, and Pursed Lip Breathing is used during acute exacerbation and End-Expiratory, Buteyko Breathing, Exhale With Activity, Stressed Respiratory Exercises,

Panting, Pacing are commonly used when the subjects are in their stable phase.

18. Breathing control is synonymous with diaphragmatic breathing. But the only difference is that in diaphragmatic breathing, it is done with maximal inspiration whereas in breathing control technique is performed at normal tidal volume. The application of breathing control technique includes its use along with FET and to control breathlessness.
19. Pursed lip breathing exercise (PLB) stresses on expiration therefore it can be used to control breathlessness and to reduce work of breathing. It keeps airways open by creating back pressure in the airways. The procedure is such that subject loosely purse the lips and exhale (like blowing out a match stick or candle). PLB decrease respiratory rate, increase tidal volume, improves exercises tolerance. It can be active and passive. PLB with forceful Expiration can increase turbulence in airways and cause further restriction.
20. Innocenti technique aimed to prevent forceful expiration thereby reduction of excess energy consumption and improves expiratory flow. Procedure is that at each breath instructs the subject to inhale just before abdominal muscle recruitment. This allows smooth transition from inspiration to expiration practice first with physiotherapist voice then without. It helps to prevent airway shutdown consumes less energy than pursed lip breathing thereby improving PaO_2.
21. End-expiratory hold mimics as that of Buteyko breathing.
22. Buteyko technique is performed by slowing respiratory rate with breath counting and at night, lying on left side and taping mouth closed. The hold at the end of expiration elevates $PaCO_2$ which helps in bronchodilatation during stable phase. This technique reverses the symptoms, lessens the need for medication and prevents asthma attacks.
23. Tension due to fear and anxiety prevents full relaxation of muscles of inspiration, therefore FRC is not attained. So stressed expiratory exercises can be given to these types of subjects. It can give also to aid clearance of secretions. Also this exercise allows identifying presence of secretions from the sounds. The unwanted side effect can be production of low lung volume. There are two types of stressed expiratory exercises.
    a. The first type is high volume high velocity where subject can do either:
        i. relaxed expiration to FRC from VC (no real forcing of expiration); or
        ii. Panting where subjects inhale to VC, briefly exhale forcefully at high lung volume, inhale to VC and repeat several times.
    b. The other type is low volume (similar to Huff) high or low velocity. In this technique subjects will inhale to VC and exhale without inhaling 3-4 times down to RV.
24. Pacing is a technique where breathing is coordinated with activity. This can decrease WOB and relieve dyspnea during activity. Subject and therapist simply test different inspiratory to expiratory ratios with various activities like cycling, walking, stair climbing until they find the rate and pattern that lower RR, relieves dyspnea and possibly improves SaO_2. For example for every two steps exhalation followed by next step with inhalation.
25. Exhale with effort is employed only in most severely impaired subjects or those with greatest complaints of dyspnea. The procedure

for this technique is to teach the subjects to break any activity into one or more breaths (bending, lifting and getting out of bed). Then Steps are: inhale during rest with Diaphragmatic breaths, Exhale through pursed lips during activity, Repeat sequence, Stopping of motion during inspiration and continuing until activity is accomplished.

26. Respiratory muscle training can be of inspiratory muscle training and expiratory muscle training. The training intensity will be the percentage of maximal inspiratory pressure for inspiratory muscle training and percentage of maximal expiratory pressure for expiratory muscle training. Inspiratory muscle training can be classified as low pressure high flow loading or high pressure low flow loading.
    a. In low pressure high flow loading also called as Normocapneic hyperpenic training increase the rate of breathing without altering $PaCO_2$ value. In this technique subjects were asked to breath at the highest rate they can manage for 15-30 minutes. A rebreathing circuit (polyethene bag, face mask) or addition of CO_2 to inspired air must be used to prevent hypocapnea. The purpose is to increase endurance of respiratory muscles.
    b. High pressure low flow loading can be of two types Inspiratory resistive training or Inspiratory threshold training:
        i. The purpose of inspiratory resistive training is that to increase strength and endurance of respiratory muscles. In this method the subject inhales through the tube of varying diameter. If diameter is narrow, there will be more resistance in the tube. First use the tube with greater diameter then gradually reduce the diameter. Limitation of this method is that load can be lessened by patients taking slow breaths to reduce turbulence (Figure 7.1).

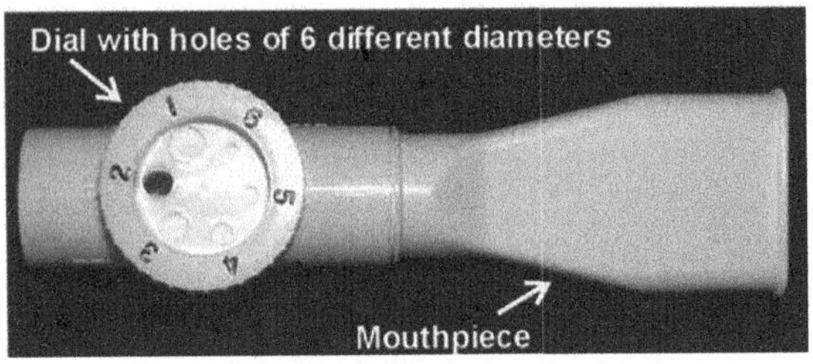

Fig. 7.1: Inspiratory resistance training

        ii. The purpose of inspiratory threshold training is same as that of inspiratory resistive training. Studies have shown that it can decrease breathlessness, increase exercise tolerance and increase nocturnal saturation. A pressure threshold device incorporates a spring loaded one-way valve, which opens to permit airflow only when a preset inspiratory pressure has been reached. The load can be a set percentage of Maximal inspiratory pressure for e.g., 80% for strength and 60% for endurance training. Patient should be trained for 5 minutes, twice a day initially later progress to three times for 15 minutes (Figure 7.2).

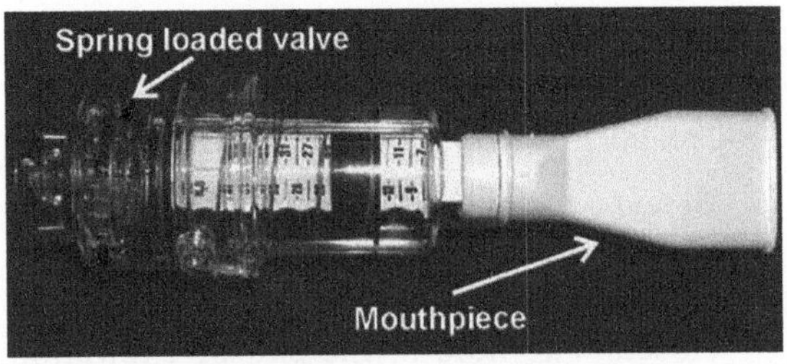

Fig. 7.2: Inspiratory threshold training

iii. In diaphragmatic training using weights mechanical resistance will be given for diaphragm muscle for the subjects with cervical and high thoracic lesions. Subject placed in supine position. Weight pan is placed over the epigastric region. Subjects with neurologically intact diaphragm can usually start with 5 pounds. If a subject begins to use sternocleido-mastoid, weight should be decreased.

27. Breathing cycle technique is used in subjects with chronic hyperventilation syndrome where there are no organic causes. Low level of CO_2 produces systemic effects such as palpitation, tachycardia, breathlessness, dysphagia, dizziness muscle pain; headache etc. In this technique there will be history of emotional disturbance. A sequence of instructions will be given. In out in out in out, in out and in out and in, In out two three in out two three, In and out two three in and out, In and out two relax hold wait in and In one two out two three four five and in one two out. The inclusion of instructions such as "and" and numbers make the patient calm down from breathlessness thereby relieving from breathlessness.

Suggested Sequence for Administering General Breathing Exercises

1. **Assessment:** Assess for any indication for breathing exercises as mentioned before.
2. **Preparation for breathing exercises:** Patient should be in relaxed position. Prior to teaching breathing exercises, perform bronchial drainage if required. The subjects can be given bronchodilators through nebulisation and humidification if required. Humidification to counteract dry atmosphere and dehydration. Analgesics may be prescribed, if pain is inhibiting deep breathing.
3. **Choice of breathing patterns:** Normally subjects predominantly use apical pattern. So stress lateral costal and diaphragmatic breathing or a combination. Unilateral breathing exercise can be given in case of lobectomy. Manual contact is given to provide extraceptive input and proprioceptive input. Also assist expiration by assisting the downward and inward movement of chest wall. In subjects with mild chronic disease or those after acute exacerbation, who are using accessory muscles, their use must be discouraged. In subjects with severe lung impairment or those with acute exacerbation, therapist should not attempt to alter the pattern.
4. **Choice of starting position:** If no dyspnoea present, position should allow for freedom by movement of diaphragm and rib cage and also allow the subject to concentrate on breathing. The arms relaxed by sides to prevent tension in thoracohumeral muscles. Lumbar spine flattened and abdominal wall relaxed as in half lying, sitting crook lying half lying. Choose position which allows for greatest excursion of diaphragm. In supine lying greater resistance of weight of abdominal viscera which may be present if subject is horizontal or tipped head down. Gravity tends to assist descend of diaphragm in the upright position but it is only capable of small excursion since it is already very low in position. In side lying, isolation of lateral costal expansion is possible for upper most lungs. Diaphragmatic breathing in side lying will preferentially distribute inspired air to dependent lung. If dyspnoea is present, ensure relaxation of abdominals by hip flexed sitting assisted by gravity the descend of diaphragm during inspiration. In forward lean sitting there will be increased activity of neck extension than neck flexors compresses viscera and pushes a low diaphragm up

enhancing its potential for improved excursion. Perfusion will be more in the upper lobes in tipped position improves V/Q matching which is helpful in pan lobular emphysema, which affects lower lobe. Lying supine flat tipped down to maximum of 15 to 20 degree puts diaphragm at higher level to improve excursion. This advantage may be counter-acted by air trapping which prevents this upward movement. But the tip of more than 20 degrees reduces this advantage even in the normal. In disease such as ascites and obesity produces more weight on the diaphragm which further reduces the disadvantage.

Chapter 8

Incentive Spirometry

HISTORY

Barlett, 1973.

INTRODUCTION

Incentive spirometer is designed to mimic natural sighing by encouraging the patients to take slow, deep breaths. Incentive spirometry is performed using device called as spirometer that provide visual cues to the patients that the desired flow or volume has been achieved.

Physiological Basis

The basic maneuver of IS is a sustained maximal inspiration (explained in previous chapter). With SMI there is drop in intrapleural pressure which increases transpulmonary pressure gradient. Greater the transpulmonary pressure gradient drop more lung expansion will occur. It also expands the lungs by boosting collateral circulation and the mechanism of physiology of interdependence.

Indications

1. Presence of pulmonary atelectasis.
2. Presence of conditions predisposing to atelectasis.
3. Upper abdominal surgery.
4. Thoracic surgery (lung and cardiac surgeries).
5. Presence of restrictive lung disorders.

TYPES

Flow Oriented Spirometer

It measure and visually indicate the degree of inspiratory flow, e.g., Triflo, Mediflo, Medciser. In the triflo device, ping pong like balls are enclosed in three connected plastic flow tubes. Each tube is calibrated such that full displacement of its ball equals a specific flow as indicated on the wall as 600 cc/sec on first tube, 900 cc/sec on the second and 1200 cc/sec on the third tube. As flow exceeds the maximum for the first tube, the ball in the second tube rises. Two out of three plastic balls should be raised and the breath sustained for some seconds while they are suspended. The third ball is a control and should not be raised because this indicates high flow and turbulence. The triflo is less encouraging for sustaining an end inspiratory hold and it is possible to cheat by taking short sharp breaths (Figures 8.1 and 8.2).

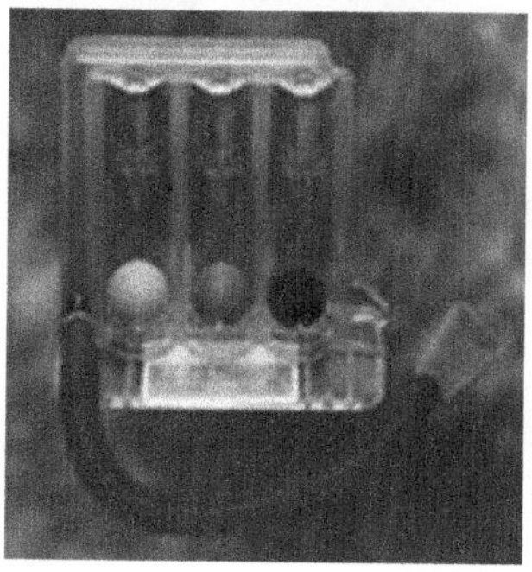

Fig. 8.1: Flow oriented spirometer: Triflo meter (See colour plate no. I)

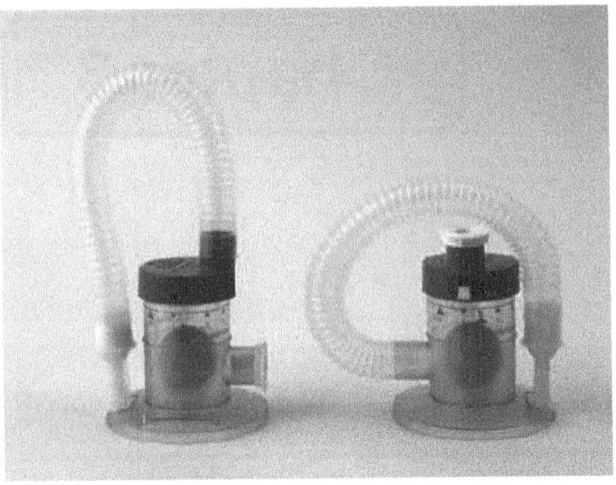

Fig. 8.2: Flow oriented spirometer: Mediflo
(See colour plate no. I)

Volume Oriented Spirometer

It actually measure and visually indicate the volume achieved during a sustained maximal inspiration, e.g., coach and volydyne. In coach and volydyne spirometer, the patient is encouraged slow and controlled inhalation by maintaining a marker (indicating flow) between two arrows and encourage an end inspiratory hold while a disc (indicating volume) moves (Figures 8.3 to 8.5).

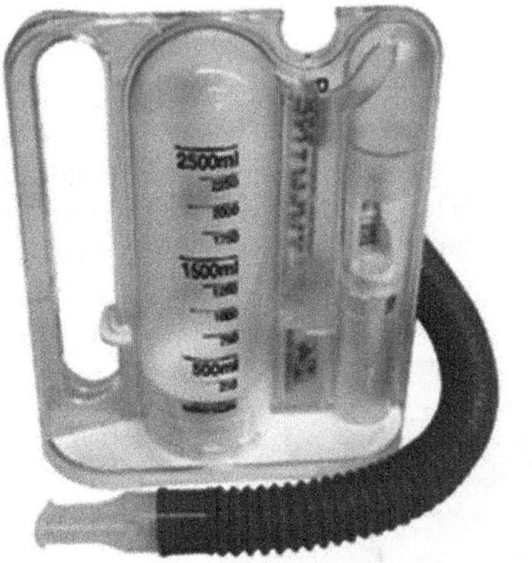

Fig. 8.3: Volume oriented spirometer:
Volydyne 2500 ml capacity
(See colour plate no. I)

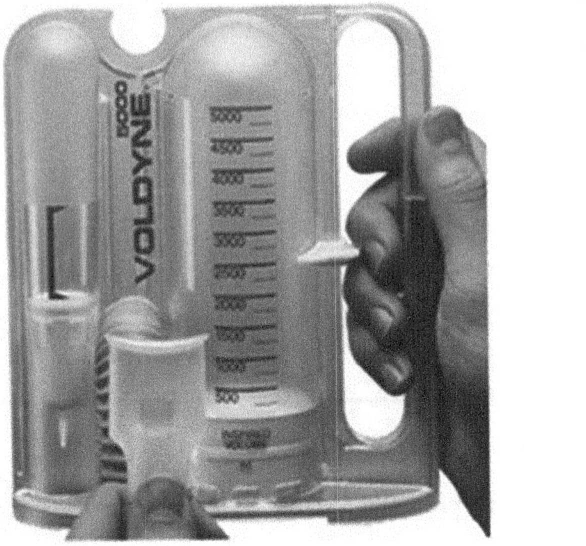

Fig. 8.4: Volume oriented spirometer:
Volydyne 5000 ml capacity
(See colour plate no. I)

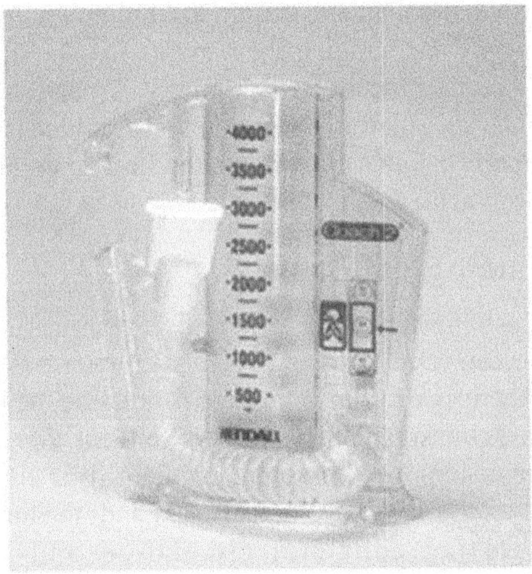

Fig. 8.5: Volume oriented spirometer: Coach spirometer
(See colour plate no. I)

Technique

The suggested technique is the following:

- Demonstration should be given to the patient by using a separate spirometer.

- Position of the patients can be half lying, side lying or high sitting.
- Patient should be relaxed prior to exercise.
- Lips should be sealed around mouthpiece then the patient inhales slowly and deeply and inspiratory hold is retained.
- Patients should be monitored throughout the procedure.
- Patients are instructed to take 10 breaths per waking hour.

Contraindications

- Unconscious patients.
- Patients who are unable to cooperate.
- Patients who cannot properly use Spirometer after instruction.
- Patient unable to generate adequate inspiration if VC < 10 mL/Kg.

Hazards and Complications

- Hyperventilation and respiratory alkalosis.
- Pulmonary barotrauma.
- Discomfort secondary to inadequate pain control.
- Hypoxemia with interruption of therapy.
- Exacerbation of bronchospasm.
- Fatigue.

Chapter 9

Mechanical Aids to Increase Lung Volume and to Reduce Work of Breathing

Continuous Positive Airway Pressure (CPAP)

INTRODUCTION

Continuous Positive Airway Pressure (CPAP) is mode of ventilation where positive pressure is given during both inspiration and expiration. It is used in both invasive and non-invasive ventilation. In non-invasive ventilation the patient breaths through face mask, nasal mask or through mouthpiece and through T piece for invasive ventilation. CPAP is administered for spontaneously breathing patients who cannot master the breath for incentive spirometer. CPAP delivers constant flow through out inspiration and expiration. This exceeds the flow rate of patients even when they are breathless. The constant pressure is set between 2.5 and 20 cm H_2O.

Effects

- Increasing the transpulmonary pressure gradient.
- Improving collateral ventilation.
- Due to physiology of interdependence.
- Increases FRC.
- Improves gas exchange.
- May avoid the need for intubation and mechanical ventilation.
- Can prevent atelectasis.
- Re-expansion of collapsed tissue (with pressure more than 15 cm H_2O).
- To reduce work of breathing in case of obstructed airways (it may relieve inspiratory muscles from their exhausting work of holding to open the obstructed airways). CPAP takes over this work during inspiration and keeps the airway open to allow greater gas emptying during expiration.

Indications

- Can be used for patients with pneumonia.
- Following major surgeries to improve gas exchange.
- As one of the weaning methods.
- Type I respiratory failure.
- A flail chest can be stabilised with CPAP.

Complications

- At high pressures, gas can be forced into stomach, causing discomfort and restricted breathing.

- Aspiration if patients unable to remove their mask rapidly.
- Coughing without removing the mask can create high pressures which may damage ear and pneumothorax.
- Machine is noisy and produces discomfort to patients and neighbours.
- Hemodynamic effects; reduced cardiac output: over distension of alveoli compresses pulmonary blood vessels this increases right ventricular afterload. Positive pressure in the thorax results in reduced venous return. Both of which reduces cardiac output.
- Carbon dioxide retention may occur if a hypercapnic patients breathes with a small tidal volume against a high pressure valve.

Contraindications

- Type II respiratory failure: Results in carbon dioxide retention.
- An un-drained pneumothorax.
- Surgical emphysema.
- Large bullae.
- Lung abscess as the size of air space may increase.
- Severe hemoptysis till it lessens.
- Facial trauma.
- Excessive secretions.

Precautions

It should be used in caution with following conditions like:

- Bronchopleural fistula.
- A large tumour in the proximal airways because air may be able to cross the obstruction but will not be able to exit.

Bi-level Positive Airway Pressure (BiPAP)

INTRODUCTION

BiPAP is mode of ventilation where positive pressure is given during both inspiration and expiration. However inspiratory pressure is more than expiratory pressure. It is used in both invasive and non-invasive ventilation. In non-invasive ventilation the patients breaths through face mask, nasal mask or through mouthpiece and through T piece for invasive ventilation. BiPAP is more comfortable than CPAP and more flexible than IPPB. It is the non-invasive equivalent of pressure support with PEEP. Inspiratory pressure is set at 10-14 cm H_2O and expiratory pressure is set at 2-4 cm H_2O. If inspiratory pressure is equal to expiratory pressure it will work as CPAP. BiPAP is flow triggered, pressure controlled and flow cycled.

Effects

- Increasing the transpulmonary pressure gradient.
- Improving collateral ventilation.
- Due to mechanism of physiology of interdependence.
- Commonly used to reduce work of breathing (mechanism explained in CPAP).
- Improve sleep.
- Reduce breathlessness.
- Improves gas exchange.
- Increases FRC.
- May avoid the need for intubation and mechanical ventilation.

Indications

- Acute exacerbation of COPD or Asthma.
- Type I respiratory failure.

- Type II respiratory failure.
- Hyperinflation of collapsed lungs.

Complications

- At high pressures, gas can be forced into stomach, causing discomfort and restricted breathing.
- Aspiration if patients unable to remove their mask rapidly.
- Coughing without removing the mask can create high pressures which may damage ear and pneumothorax.
- Machine is noisy and produces discomfort to patients and neighbours.
- Hemodynamic effects; reduced cardiac output: Overdistension of alveoli compresses pulmonary blood vessels this increases right ventricular afterload. Positive pressure in the thorax results in reduced venous return. Both of which reduces cardiac output.

Contraindications

- An un-drained pneumothorax.
- Surgical emphysema.
- Facial trauma.
- Excessive secretions.

Precautions

It should be used in caution with following conditions like:

- Bronchopleural fistula.
- A large tumour in the proximal airways because air may be able to cross the obstruction but will not be able to exit.

Intermittent Positive Pressure Breathing (IPPB)

INTRODUCTION

Intermittent positive pressure breathing is non-invasive ventilation where positive pressure is administered during ventilation which is intermittent. The patient can breath through face mask or nasal mask. It is pressure supported ventilation where inspiration is triggered by the patient, sustained by positive pressure and followed by passive expiration. Inspiratory pressure sensitivity (triggering the breath), flow rate and inspiratory pressure are three settings in this type of ventilator. There will be also air-mix knob for setting FiO_2 and apnea switch which controls automatic function and work as ventilator. IPPB is administered for semi-conscious patients. It has some disadvantages compared to other mechanical aids. It is less effective than spontaneous deep breathing that's why IPPB is unnecessary for patients who can breathe independently. The extra volume is distributed preferentially to areas already well ventilated. Hence position the collapsed lung uppermost during the administration of IPPB.

Effects

- Increasing the transpulmonary pressure gradient.
- Improving collateral ventilation.
- Due to the mechanism of physiology of interdependence.
- Increases lung volume (CPAP increases FRC whereas IPPB increases tidal volume).
- Improve ventilation.
- Improves gas exchange.
- To reduce work of breathing (mechanism explained in CPAP).
- It clears out secretion by inducing passive cough reflux.

Indications

- Patients with atelectasis.
- For sputum retention.
- To reduce work of breathing.
- Whenever the patient is exhausted.

- Type II respiratory failure.
- To deliver Entonox (mixture of nitrous oxide and oxygen) for pain relief.

Complications

- **Air swallowing occurs:** This may be showed by cheek distension and burping. This may be relieved by left side lying.
- Hypercapnic COPD patients may lose their hypoxic respiratory drive because of oxygen delivery with IPPB.
- **Hemodynamic effects; reduced cardiac output:** Overdistension of alveoli compresses pulmonary blood vessels this increases right ventricular afterload. Positive pressure in the thorax results in reduced venous return. Both of which reduces cardiac output.
- Carbon dioxide retention may occur if a hypercapnic patient breathes with a small tidal volume against a high pressure valve.

Contraindications

- An un-drained pneumothorax.
- Surgical emphysema.
- Large bullae.
- Lung abscess as the size of air space may increase.
- Severe hemoptysis till it lessens facial trauma.

Precautions

It should be used in caution with following conditions like:

- Bronchopleural fistula.
- A large tumour in the proximal airways because air may be able to cross the obstruction but will not be able to exit.

Chapter 10

Positive Airway Pressure (PAP) Adjuncts

Positive airway pressure adjuncts include the use of PEP, Flutter, Acapella, CPAP and EPAP to mobilize secretions and treat atelectasis.

PEP Therapy

INTRODUCTION

Positive expiratory pressure therapy is the application of positive pressure at the mouth during expiration. In this therapy positive pressure is generated as the patient exhales through a **fixed orifice resistor**, generating pressures ranging from 10 to 120 cm H_2O. Fixed orifice resistor generates pressure only when expired flows are high enough to generate back pressure through the small orifice.

Parts

Consists of mask or mouthpiece connected to one way breathing valve to which expiratory resistors are attached. This results in positive pressure in airways (Figure 10.1).

Types

High PEP: 50 to 120 cm H_2O, applied only during slight active expiration.

Low PEP: 10 to 20 cm H_2O.

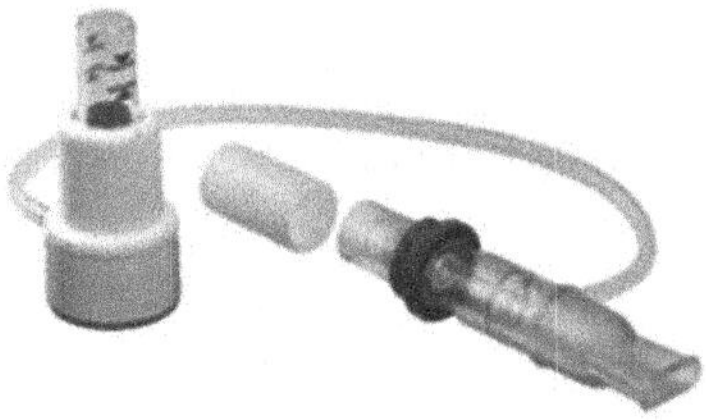

Fig. 10.1: PEP

Indications

Indications are described in the Box 10.1.

Box 10.1: Indications of PEP, Flutter and Acapella
1. To reduce air trapping in asthma and COPD 2. To aid in mobilization of retained secretions (in cystic fibrosis and chronic bronchitis) 3. To prevent or reverse atelectasis 4. To optimize delivery of bronchodilators 5. To reduce the incidence of chest infections

Principles of Operation

When the patients breathe out through PEP, back pressure is created which forces air through collateral channels. This moves the mucus plug more central (towards trachea) and boost mucociliary clearance (Figure 10.2).

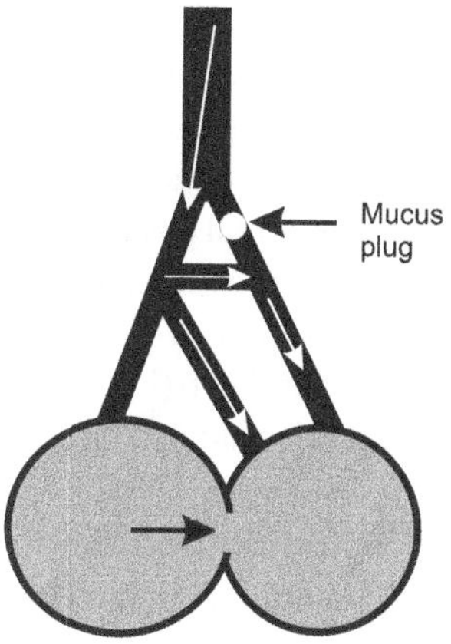

Fig. 10.2: Mechanism of PEP therapy

Technique

Patient sits leaning forward with elbows supported on a table. Mouthpiece/mask can be used. Patient inhales normally (or at greater than normal tidal volume, but less than total lung capacity). The smallest diameter (child: 1.5 mm and adult 2.5-3.5 mm) is chosen which the patient can use comfortably for two minutes to achieve a pressure 12-15 cm H_2O. Patient exhales actively, but not forcefully, against fixed-orifice resistor. As the secretions move centrally, breaths can be taken at higher tidal volumes. Exhalation should not last more than 4 seconds. Monitoring the manometer is done by physiotherapist rather than patient otherwise patient may alter breathing pattern. Breathing cycle is repeated 10 - 20 times interspersed with relaxed breaths. When secretions are mobilised, patient performs several forced expiratory maneuvers (Huff cough) or ACBT or AD to clear the secretions.

Contraindications

There are no absolute contraindications.

- Patients unable to tolerate the increased work of breathing.
- Hemodynamic instability.
- Intracranial pressure (ICP) > 20 mm Hg.
- Recent facial, oral, or skull surgery or trauma.
- Acute sinusitis.
- Epistaxis.
- Esophageal surgery.
- Active hemoptysis.
- Nausea.
- Known or suspected tympanic membrane rupture or other middle ear pathology.
- Untreated pneumothorax.

Hazards/Complications

- Increased work of breathing that may lead to hypoventilation and hypercarbia.
- Increased intracranial pressure.
- Cardiovascular compromise:
  - Myocardial ischemia.
  - Decreased venous return.
- Air swallowing, with increased likelihood of vomiting and aspiration.
- Skin breaks down and discomfort from mask
- Pulmonary barotrauma.

Flutter Valve Therapy

INTRODUCTION

Flutter is a device resembling short broad pipe which produces positive oscillatory pressure of 10-20 cm H_2O. Oscillations are caused by vibrations of steel ball within the cone (Figure 10.3).

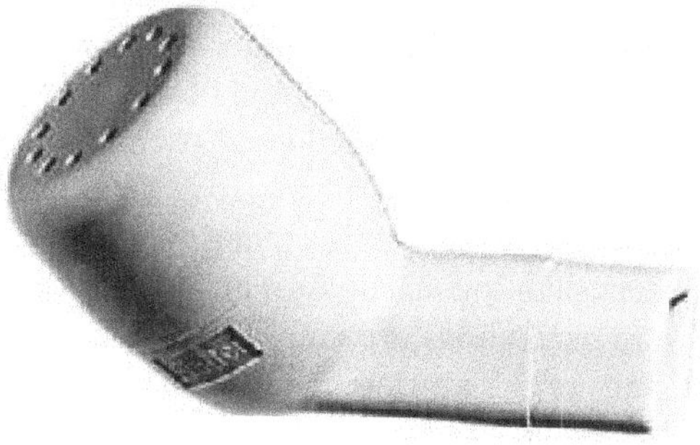

Fig. 10.3: Flutter

Parts

- Mouthpiece.
- High density steel ball.
- Circular cone.
- Perforated protective cover (Figure 10.4).

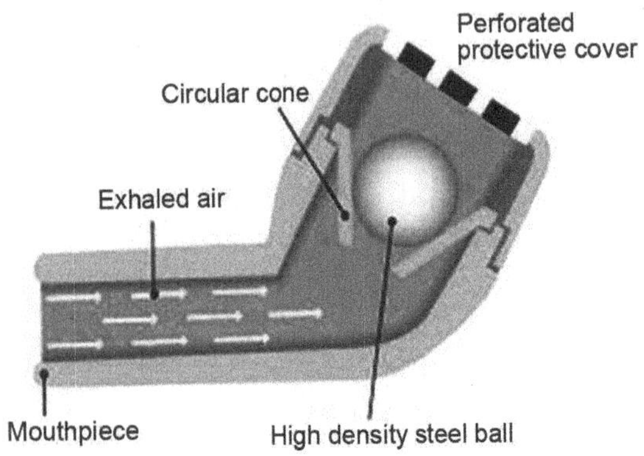

Fig. 10.4: Flutter parts

Principle of Operation

It is based on its ability to:

- Vibrate the airways.
- Intermittently increase endobronchial pressure.
- Accelerate expiratory airflow.

Before exhalation, the steel ball blocks the conical canal of the flutter. During exhalation, the actual position of the steel ball is the result of equilibrium between: (1) the pressure of the exhaled air, (2) the force of gravity on the ball, and (3) the angle of the cone where the contact with the ball occurs. As the steel ball rolls and bounces up and down, it results in production of oscillations in expiratory pressure and airflow. When the oscillation frequency approximates the resonance frequency of the pulmonary system, endobronchial pressure oscillations are amplified and result in vibrations of the airways. The flutter produces a range of oscillation frequencies between 6 and 20 Hz, which corresponds to the range of the pulmonary resonance frequencies in humans. Attaining oscillation frequencies in this range is fundamental to the efficacy of the flutter. The oscillation frequency produced by the flutter when its stem is in the horizontal position is approximately 15 Hz. This frequency can be modulated by changing the inclination of the flutter slightly up (higher frequency) or down (lower frequency) from its original horizontal position. This is called as tilting.

Indications

Indications are mentioned in the Box 10.1.

Effects

When correctly, the effect is 3-fold:

1. Vibrations applied to the airway facilitate the loosening of secretions.
2. The increase in bronchial pressure helps avoid air trapping.
3. Expiratory air flows are accelerated and facilitate the upward movement of mucus.

Technique

Position of the patient: The patient should be seated with back straight and head slightly tilted upward so the upper airway is wide open. This will allow exhaled air to flow smoothly from the lungs and out through the flutter. To adjust the flutter to the patient's pulmonary resonance. Move the flutter slightly up or down to achieve the maximum "fluttering" effect. This resonance is evidenced by the vibrations that can be felt within the chest by the patients or by observation or palpation by the therapist.

Stage 1: Mucus Loosening and Mucus Mobilization

Instruct the patient to slowly inhale to approximately 3/4 of a full breath. Position the flutter at the proper angle and perform a 2 to 3 second breath-hold. The patient should exhale through the flutter at a reasonably fast but not too forceful speed. Continue to exhale to a level slightly further than one would exhale during normal breathing without the flutter. Repeat this breathing technique for another 5 to 10 breaths. The mucus moves further up the airways with each flutter exhalation. The angle at which the patient holds the flutter is critical. Initially stem is horizontal to the floor, which places the cone at a slight tilt. Tilt insures that the ball not only bounces but also rolls during exhalation. Emphasize the patients to hold the breath 2 to 3 seconds, and suppressing the urge to cough.

Stage 2: Mucus Elimination

Breath in slowly and fully as comfortably possible and followed by 2 to 3 seconds breath-hold. Exhale forcefully and completely throughout the flutter. The forceful exhalation moves mucus up to a level in the lungs that triggers a cough. If the mucus is not easily coughed out following 1 or 2 elimination breaths, attempt a "huff" maneuver. Series of 5 to 10 mucus loosening breaths with cough suppression followed by 1 or 2 mucus elimination breaths with cough should result in successful airway clearance. Clean the device on a regular basis by disassembling and soaking.

Contraindications

Patients with pneumothorax or overt right-sided heart failure.

Hazards and Complications

Same as that of PEP.

Acapella

INTRODUCTION

Acapella is similar to PEP but adds vibration therapy as well. It is always delivered with aerosol therapy. Acapella is a small hand-held device that combines the resistive features of a PEP valve and the vibratory features of a flutter valve to mobilize secretions in the airway. It uses a counterweighted plug and magnet directs exhaled air through a pivoting cone, to generate airflow vibrations between 0-30 Hz. Both the vibration frequencies and the resistive pressures are adjustable.

Types of Acapella Models

The acapella is available in two color-coded models. The green acapella is suitable for patients able to maintain an expiratory flow of 15 LPM or greater for 3 seconds and the blue acapella is suitable for the patients who are not capable of maintaining 15 LPM flow for 3 seconds (Figure 10.5).

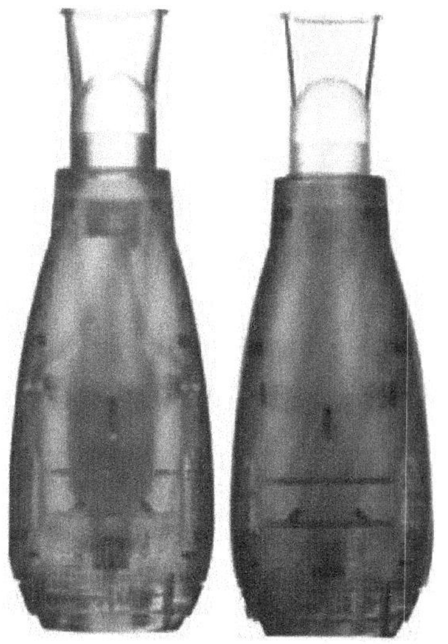

Fig. 10.5: Acapella (See colour plate no. I)

Procedure

Initial Settings

With the first use of acapella, ensure that the frequency adjustment dial is turned counter-clockwise to the lowest frequency-resistance setting. For frequency/resistance increase dial has to turn clockwise. To provide simultaneous aerosol drug delivery, attach nebulizer to the end of the acapella. Place mouthpiece lightly in mouth; maintain a tight seal on the mouthpiece during inspiration. Patient has to be relaxed while performing diaphragmatic breathing. Inspire a volume of air which should be greater than tidal volume, but less than total lung capacity. Instruct patient to slowly inhale to 3/4 maximum breathing capacity. Instruct the patient to hold breath for 2-3 seconds. Direct the patient to exhale to functional residual capacity (FRC) actively, but not too forcefully, through the device. Emphasize the patient for breath-holding, and suppressing the urge to cough. The patient should be able to exhale for 3-4 seconds while the device vibrates. If the patient cannot maintain an exhalation for this length of time, adjust the dial clockwise. Clockwise adjustment increases the resistance of the vibrating orifice, which will allow the patient to exhale at a lower flow-rate. Perform the technique for 10-20 breaths.

Contraindications, hazards and complications same as that of PEP.

Home exercise to clear secretions without any devices:

"Blow Bottle Exercise"

A 50 cm plastic tube (1 cm diameter) is put in a bottle containing 10 cm of water. Patient was asked to blow through the tube. This will clear out secretions.

Chapter 11

Coughing and Huffing Techniques

DEFINITION

Coughing is an expiratory effort with a closed glottis.

Stages of Coughing

A cough stimulus is initiated by irritation of trachea. By irritation an abnormal stimulus provokes sensory fibres in the airways to send impulses to the brain's medullary cough center. The stimulus normally is mechanical, chemical, thermal or inflammation. Foreign bodies can provoke a cough through mechanical stimulation. Chemical stimulation can occur when irritating gases are inhaled (smoking). Infection is a good example of cough stimulation due to an inflammatory process. Finally, cold air may cause thermal stimulation of sensory nerves and produce a cough.

According to Linder, a cough reflux has four stages which are mentioned as follows:

1. Deep Inspiration

Once the impulses are received, the cough center generates a reflex stimulation of the respiratory muscles to initiate a deep inspiration. This stage provides the volume necessary for a forceful cough. At least 60% Predicted Vital capacity should achieve for an effective coughing.

2. Closure of Glottis

The reflux nerve impulses causes glottis closure. This is achieved by closure of Vocal Folds. This prepares the abdominal and intercostal muscles to produce positive intrathoracic pressure distal to glottis (> 100 mm of Hg).

3. Forceful Contraction of Abdominal Muscles

Contraction of abdominal and intercostals muscles lasts for 0.2 seconds. This phase results in a rapid rise in pleural and alveolar pressures.

4. Opening of Glottis and Forceful Exhalation

When the glottis is open a large pressure gradient is established between the alveoli and the airway opening. Along with contraction of expiratory muscles, this pressure gradient causes a violent expulsive flow of air from the lungs.

High velocity gas flow combined with dynamic airway compression creates huge shear forces that displace mucous from the airway walls into the air stream.

Evaluation of Coughing

Position: Ask the patient to assume the posture,

he adopts for coughing. To see the patients coughing pattern ask the patient to demonstrate the cough.

Then coughing has to be evaluated stage-wise:

Stage 1

Look for spontaneous inspiration.

Use of trunk movements such as extension of neck, trunk etc.

Eye Gaze: An upward gaze is good for effective pattern.

Stage 2

Glottis closure has to be evaluated.

Ask the patient to hold his breath if you hear a cough then the patient is not able to close the glottis.

Stage 3

In this stage active contraction of abdominal muscles has to be observed.

Throaty cough indicates cough is with inadequate force.

Stage 4

During expulsion does the patient appear to gag before successfully allowing air to exhale has to be noted?

Instruction to Facilitate Coughing

Instructions can be given stage-wise to facilitate coughing.

Stage 1

Verbal cues and positioning can be given to enhance inspiration.

Active arm movements like flexion or abduction can be used to increase the inspiration.

Following commands will be effective to facilitate the stage 1:

- Look upward while inhale.
- Raise both arms up.
- Squeeze your shoulders back while you inhale.
- Extend your back while inhale.

Stage 2

In stage 2 glottis closure is necessary. Verbal cues such as deep breath and hold the breath will help to improve the closure of glottis. Practice of stacked breathing exercises, deep breathing with inspiratory hold and airshift breathing will improve the control of closure of glottis.

Stage 3

Pain relieving maneuvers such as application of intense TENS or administration of analgesics can help in forceful contraction of abdominal muscles.

Following commands will be effective to facilitate the stage 3:

- Look down while you cough.
- Pull both of the arms down to your hip.
- Bend your neck and back while you exhale.

Stage 4

Forceful expulsion of air can be facilitated by self-assisted or therapist assisted techniques.

Prior to coughing patient should be well hydrated. Humidification is required if upper air-way is bypassed or if patient is on oxygen therapy. Patient should also be nebulised based prior to coughing. This can be bland aerosol therapy or therapeutic aerosol therapy.

Coughing Techniques

Coughing techniques are classified into active, passive, assisted coughing techniques (Flowchart 11.1).

Active Coughing Techniques

Following are the types of active coughing techniques:

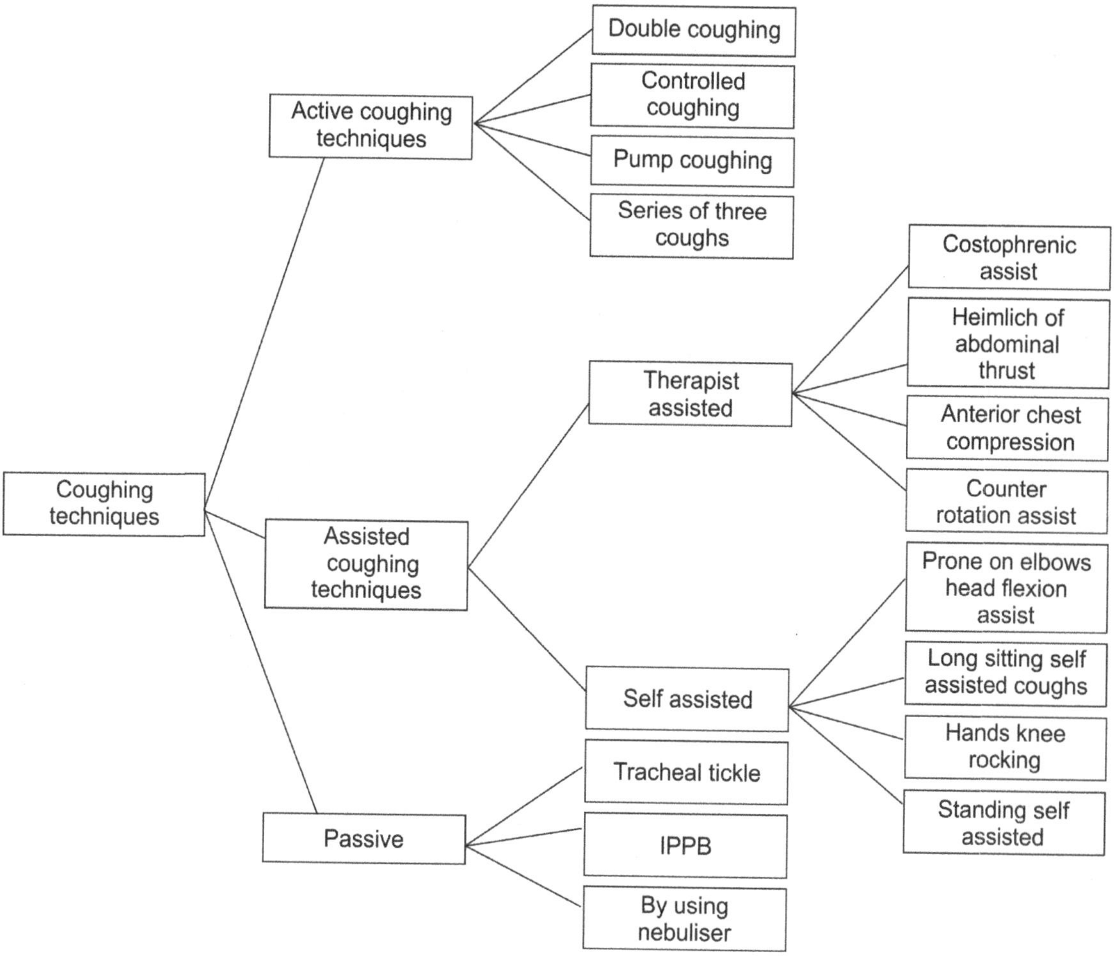

Flowchart 11.1: Classification of coughing techniques

1. **Double Coughing:** Following deep inspiration patient performs two coughs in one breath. Second is more forceful than first.
2. **Controlled Coughing:** Patient takes three deep breaths exhaling normally after first two and then coughing firmly on third. The first two breaths are believed to decrease atelectasis and increase volume of cough.
3. **Pump Coughing:** The patient take deep breaths and then gives three short easy coughs followed by three huffs. This facilitates secretion clearance in patients with air trapping (emphysema).
4. **Series of Three Coughs:** The patient take a small breath, gives a fair cough then a bigger breath gives a harder cough and finally a really deep breath and gives a forceful cough. It is used for post-operative patients.

Passive Coughing Techniques

Here the patient does not have any role in initiating a cough. Any of the following technique is used to produce a cough reflux:

1. **Tracheal tickle:** Used for patients coming out of anesthesia.

2. **A suction effort** may produce coughing effort.
3. **IPPB.**
4. **Nebuliser.**
5. **Hydration with warm water.**

Assisted Coughing Techniques

In this type of coughing techniques either therapist hands or patient themselves uses their hands to assist coughing. It is divided into manual assisted coughing technique where therapist hands are used in assisting or self assisted where patients themselves assist cough with their hands.

Manually Assisted Techniques

Prior to perform techniques; give instructions to the patient to maximise four stages of coughing. The patient also actively participates by using his or her arms, trunk, or other body parts throughout the entire procedure.

1. Costophrenic Assist

Position the patient mostly in sitting or side lying; the therapist places his or her hands on the costophrenic angles of the rib cage. At the end of the patient's next exhalation, the therapist applies a quick manual stretch down and in toward the patient's navel to facilitate a stronger diaphragmatic and intercostals muscle contraction during the succeeding inhalation. Just a moment before asking the patient to actively cough, the therapist applies strong pressure through his or her hands, again down and in toward the navel. In this manner the therapist is assisting both the build up of intrathoracic pressure and the force of expiration.

2. Heimlich-type Assist or Abdominal Thrust Assist

The therapist places the heel of his or her hand at about the level of the patient's navel. As the patient is instructed to cough, the therapist quickly pushes up and in, under the diaphragm with the heel of his or her hand, as in a Heimlich choking manoeuvre. This procedure is very effective at forcefully expelling the air. But it can be extremely uncomfortable for the patient because of (1) its concentrated area of contact, (2) the abrupt nature, which may elicit an undesired high neuromuscular tone response or worse when combined with sensory input that the therapist's manual contacts supply, (3) the force, which may cause an abdominal herniation. Patients with low neuromuscular tone or flaccid abdominal muscles do best with this procedure.

3. Anterior Chest Compression Assist

This technique compresses both the upper and lower anterior chest during the coughing manoeuvre. The therapist puts one arm across the patient's pectoralis region to compress the upper chest and the other arm is either placed parallel on the lower chest or abdomen or placed like in the Heimlich type of manoeuvre. The therapist then applies a quick force through both arms to simulate the force necessary during the expulsion phase. The directions of the force are: (1) down and back on the upper chest, and (2) up and back on the lower chest or abdominal arm. Performed together the compression force from both arms makes the letter V.

4. Counter-Rotation Assist

Position the patient in side lying. Therapist positioned the hand over the shoulder and pelvis. The therapist assists in inhalation and exhalation and trunk rotation is performed along with inspiration and expiration. Assume the patient is on left side lying. During inspiratory phase therapist left hand is placed on patient's right scapula and right hand anterior to patient's iliac crest. As hand pushes scapula, pulling the pelvis back, greater inspiration occurs. During expiration the therapist left hand glides over the patients shoulder to reach chest and right hand glides to the patients right gluteal fossa. The therapist compresses the rib cage by pulling the shoulder back and while pushing the hip forwards.

Self-Assisted Techniques

Please note that supine position is not used for increasing lung volume or not used in any of the coughing techniques. Prone is not frequently used as a posture for coughing because the position itself inhibits full use of the diaphragm by preventing lower anterior chest and abdominal excursion following a neurologic insult. This forces the patient to use an alternate breathing pattern that facilitates greater accessory muscle use. Following are self-assisted coughing techniques mainly used in neurological patients.

1. Prone on Elbows Head Flexion Self-assisted Cough

In this technique, the patient is positioned in prone on elbows position. The therapist instructs the patient to extend his or her neck and lift the head upwards while inhaling maximally. The therapist then tells the patient to cough as the patient bends his neck downward into a completely flexed posture. Since full use of the diaphragm is not used, the resultant cough will be weaker than in other postures. After mastering the timing of the procedure, most patients move back to another posture usually sitting or side lying, and to other techniques. For the population of patients who can assume a prone on elbows posture independently (i.e., some patients with tetraplegia), this technique may be used functionally. Here, they can assist their own coughs when the need arises, rather than wait for someone to assist them in a position change.

2. Long-Sitting Self-assisted Cough

In this long-sitting self-assist technique, the patient is positioned on a mat in a long-sitting posture with upper extremity support. The therapist instructs the patient to extend his or her body backward while inhaling maximally. The therapist then tells the patient to cough as the patient throws his or her upper body forward into a completely flexed posture, using shoulder internal rotation if possible. Here the extension aspect of the procedure is used to maximize inhalation, whereas the flexion aspect is used to maximize expiration. This technique is commonly taught to tetraplegics.

3. Short-Sitting Self-assisted Cough

This technique is typically performed in a wheel chair over the edge of a bed. The patient is instructed to place one hand over the other at the wrist and place them in his or her lap. Then the patient is then asked to extend his trunk backward while inhaling maximally, followed by a strong voluntary cough. During the cough, the patient pulls his or her hands up and under the diaphragm, resembling the motion of a Heimlich maneuver. The hands mimic the abdominal muscles, which would ordinarily contract to push the intestinal contents up and under the diaphragm to aid its recoil ability. It is an effective self-assisted method for patients who have weak diaphragms or abdominal musculature like SCI or spina bifida patients with C5 or below lesions. As tetraplegics usually require trunk support they cannot perform this technique whereas most paraplegics can perform it from an unsupported short-sitting position. Patients who lack good upper-extremity coordination, such as many Parkinson's and multiple sclerosis (MS) patients, cannot perform the procedure quickly or forcefully enough to make it effective and usually require assistance from another person.

4. Hands-Knees Rocking Self-assisted Cough

This coughing technique increases patient's balance, strength and coordination along with coughing. The patient assumes an all-fours position (hand-knees). Then the patient is instructed to rock forward, looking up and breathing in as he or she moves to a fully extended posture. After this, the patient is told to cough out as he or she quickly rocks backward to the heels with a flexed head and neck. Patients with generalized or spotty weakness throughout (e.g., some SCI, head traumas, Parkinson's, MS, cerebral palsy, or spina bifida patients), this method is perfect for incorporating many functional goals into a single activity.

5. Standing Self-assisted Cough

Standing uses the same concepts and can be readily used for self-assisted coughs, provided the patient has adequate standing balance and/or upper extremity support. Combinations of trunk, head, and extremity movements, during the cough maneuver is almost endless, thus specific techniques are not itemized.

Cough Splinting or Cough Hold

INTRODUCTION

Supporting the incision while patient performs a cough effort either by himself or by physiotherapist with hands or pillows.

Indications

Commonly done for:

A. Cardiac surgeries.

B. Thoracic surgeries (Thoracotomy).

C. Abdominal surgeries.

D. Pelvic surgeries.

Splinting can be done in three ways:

- Self assisted.
- Therapist assisted.
- With the help of rib belt.

Positions for Cough Splinting

Patient should be brought to long sitting positions from half lying position with the help of nurse and physiotherapist in case of Thoracotomy and cardiac surgeries. Patient finds it easier to cough while sitting forward in bed away from pillow. A high sitting position is adopted for the patients in wards and home.

Ways of Splinting

In Case of Abdominal Surgeries

Self Assisted

A pillow or bed sheet supported by dominant hand and reinforced by non-dominant hand.

Therapist Assisted

For a laparotomy incision the patient should be high sitting position. The therapist stands behind the patient. Hands are reached towards the incision. Gentle firm pressure is directed at holding the wound edges together.

In Case of Pelvic Surgeries

Self Assisted

Thighs should be adducted, by keeping a pillow in between thigh press the thighs each other. Incision is supported by dominant hand followed by non-dominant hand.

Therapist Assisted

Same as above but therapist support the incision:

In Case of Thoracotomy

Self Assisted

Patient places the hand of the unaffected side as far round the affected ribs as possible and applying firm pressure with the hand and forearm. The other hand reinforces the hugging hold by clasping the opposite elbow and pulling it against the chest wall during the cough.

Therapist Assisted

1. *Bear hug hold:* The anterior and posterior aspects of the affected side of the thorax can be supported with the hands, while at the same time the forearm will stabilize the whole chest and create a bear hug hold. In this hold the physiotherapist holds from the opposite side.

2. Physiotherapist can hold from same side also. In this method therapist place hand anterior and posterior to the incision. Therapist applies firm pressure with the hand.

In case of Sternotomy

Self Assisted

1. Holding both hands across sternum and placing a pillow between hand and anterior portion of chest.
2. Place a small pillow over the incision and then the pillow is supported by dominant hand followed by non-dominant hand.

Therapist Assisted

1. Physiotherapist support the incision by placing both hands on the anterior aspect of the chest and maintaining equal pressure to minimise sternal movement.
2. Place dominant hand over the sternotomy incision and other hand over the back (same like bear hug hold). Patient is bought to lean forward, vibration is given through back hand and incision is supported during coughing.

Complications of Coughing

- Bronchospasm.
- Tussive syncopy.

Huffing Techniques

Huff is a rapid forced exhalation but not with maximal effort. The patient take deep inspiration and then air is forcefully exhaled as in coughing except that mouth is kept open. For, e.g., fogging a pair of eye glasses with warm breath. Rate of expiratory flow varies with individual, disease and degree of air flow obstruction. Table 11.1 differentiates effective huffing and ineffective huffing.

Table 11.1 Effective huffing and Ineffective huffing

Effective Huffing	*Ineffective Huffing*
Mouth open	Mouth half or almost closed
Muscles of chest wall and abdominals contract	Abdominal muscles not used
Sound is like sigh but forced	Sound like hissing or blowing Catching or grunting at back of throat
Rate of expiratory flow varies with individual, disease and degree of air flow obstruction	Incorrect quality of expiration Too vigorous long Too gentle Too short

Huffing can be high or low by shifting the equal pressure point towards centre or periphery. Further points are detailed in the chapter 16 ACBT.

Chapter 12

Postural Drainage Therapy

Postural drainage therapy includes turning, postural drainage, manual techniques and coughing.

DEFINITION

Postural drainage is an airway clearance technique that uses gravity to assist in the mobilisation of secretions from bronchopulmonary segments to the central airways. It is often coupled with chest physiotherapy.

Principle

Bronchopulmonary segment and its bronchus is parallel to carina in a particular position so that gravity can assist in mobilisation of secretions.

Goals

- To prevent accumulation of secretions.
- To remove secretions already accumulated.

Settings

- Critical care.
- In-patient acute care.
- Extended care and skilled nursing facility care.
- Home care.
- Outpatient/ambulatory care.
- Pulmonary diagnostic (bronchoscopy) laboratory.

Types

True postural drainage is given for the patients who are stable and exact head down positions are given to the patient. Modified postural drainage is given for the patients who are not stable that means acute exacerbation of COPD and asthma. Home postural drainage is administered in home with pillows, bean bag etc.

Equipments Required

1. *For Hospitalized Patients*
    - Bed with manual or electric devices to position the patient.
    - Air therapy beds.
    - Tilt table.
    - Pillows.
2. *For Home Treatments*
    - Pillows.
    - Slant board.
    - Foam wedge.
    - Sofa cushions.

- Chair which is inverted.
- Bean bag.
- Stacks of newspaper.

Indications

1. Indications for Turning

a. Inability or reluctance of patient to change body position (e.g., mechanical ventilation, neuromuscular disease, drug-induced paralysis).

b. Poor oxygenation associated with position (e.g., unilateral lung disease).

c. Potential for or presence of atelectasis.

d. Presence of artificial airway.

2. Indications for Postural Drainage

a. Evidence or suggestion of difficulty with secretion clearance.

b. Difficulty clearing secretions with expectorated sputum production greater than 25-30 mL/day (adult).

c. Evidence or suggestion of retained secretions in the presence of an artificial airway.

d. Presence of atelectasis caused by or suspected of being caused by mucus plugging.

e. Patients who are on prolonged bed rest.

f. Post-surgical patients who have received general anaesthesia and who may have painful incisions that restrict deep breathing and coughing post operatively.

g. Any patient who is on ventilator if they are stable enough to tolerate the patient.

h. Diagnosis of diseases such as cystic fibrosis, bronchiectasis or cavitating lung disease, chronic bronchitis, pneumonia, acute lung infections.

i. Presence of foreign body in airway.

3. Indications for External Manipulation of the Thorax

a. Sputum volume or consistency suggesting a need for additional manipulation (e.g., percussion and/or vibration) to assist movement of secretions by gravity, in a patient receiving postural drainage.

Preparation for Postural Drainage

- Hydration should be done prior to PD to reduce viscosity.
- Nebulisation of bronchodilators prior to PD.
- Familiar with bed movement for Trendelenburg position.
- Familiar with IV lines, leads, tubes attach to the patient.
- Have suctioning equipment ready and should be nearby to the patients bed.
- Never administer PD after a meal.
- Appropriate time of PD can be in early morning or late evening.
- Sputum cup availability.

Technique/Procedure

- Auscultation.
- Position the patient.
- Make the patient comfortable in the position.
- Maintain for 5 to 10 minutes.
- Monitor for saturation, pulse, arrhythmia.
- Patient should be encouraged to take deep breaths and cough after positions.
- Instruction to patient that secretions may be mobilized after one hour of treatment.
- Most affected area drain first.

Contraindications

Positioning: A in bracket stands for absolute contraindications.

1. *All positions are contraindicated for:*
   - Intracranial pressure (ICP) > 20 mm Hg.
   - Head and neck injury until stabilized (A).
   - Active hemorrhage with hemodynamic instability (A).
   - Recent spinal surgery (e.g., laminectomy) or acute spinal injury.
   - Acute spinal injury or active hemoptysis.
   - Empyema.
   - Bronchopleural fistula.
   - Pulmonary edema.
   - Congestive heart failure.
   - Large pleural effusions, pneumothorax.
   - Pulmonary embolism.
   - Aged, confused, or anxious patients who do not tolerate position changes.
   - Rib fracture, with or without flail chest.
   - Surgical wound or healing tissue.
   - Recent myocardial infarction.
2. *Trendelenburg position is contraindicated for:*
   - Intracranial pressure (ICP) > 20 mm Hg.
   - Patients in whom increased intracranial pressure is to be avoided (e.g., neurosurgery, aneurysms, eye surgery).
   - Uncontrolled hypertension.
   - Distended abdomen.
   - Esophageal surgery.
   - Recent gross hemoptysis related to recent lung carcinoma treated surgically or with radiation therapy.
   - Uncontrolled airway at risk for aspiration (tube feeding or recent meal).
   - Reverse Trendelenburg is contraindicated in the presence of hypotension or vasoactive medication.

HAZARDS

1. *Hypoxemia*

Action to Be Taken/Possible Intervention: Administer higher oxygen concentrations during procedure if potential for or observed hypoxemia exists. If patient becomes hypoxemic during treatment, administer 100% oxygen, stop therapy immediately, return patient to original resting position, and consult physician. Ensure adequate ventilation. Hypoxemia during postural drainage may be avoided in unilateral lung disease by placing the involved lung uppermost with patient on his or her side.

2. *Increased Intracranial Pressure*

Action to Be Taken/Possible Intervention: Stop therapy, return patient to original resting position, and consult physician.

3. *Acute Hypotension During Procedure*

Action to Be Taken/Possible Intervention: Stop therapy, return patient to original resting position, and consult physician.

4. *Pulmonary Hemorrhage*

Action to Be Taken/Possible Intervention: Stop therapy, return patient to original resting position, call physician immediately. Administer oxygen and maintain an airway until physician responds.

5. *Pain or Injury to Muscles, Ribs or Spine*

Action to Be Taken/Possible Intervention: Stop therapy that appears directly associated with pain or problem, exercise care in moving patient, and consult physician.

6. *Vomiting and Aspiration*

Action to Be Taken/Possible Intervention: Stop therapy, clear airway and suction as needed, administer oxygen, maintain airway, return patient to previous resting position, and contact physician immediately.

7. *Bronchospasm*

Action to Be Taken/Possible Intervention: Stop therapy, return patient to previous resting position, administer or increase oxygen delivery while contacting physician. Administer physician-ordered bronchodilators.

8. *Dysrhythmias*

Action to Be Taken/Possible Intervention: Stop therapy, return patient to previous resting position, administer or increase oxygen delivery while contacting physician.

Advantages

- Easy to learn.
- Postural drainage positions can be coordinated with other activities (for e.g., in hospital, positioning for skin pressure relief. In home such as reading or watching television.
- Cost is minimal.

Disadvantages

- Optimal positions are contraindicated in most of the conditions.
- Compliance of PD may be reduced because of the length of treatment, in case of pediatrics.

Modified Postural Drainage

Sometimes true postural drainage cannot be given in some conditions because they may develop some complications for, e.g., patients with congestive heart failure may develop orthopnea, Neurosurgery patients ICP may be increased, Post Thoracic/post cardiac surgery patients drainage tubes may limit positioning. In this case modified postural drainage is adopted. For draining lower lobes a pillow under the pelvis in supine may drain anterior basal segments and a pillow under pelvis in prone lying may drain posterior basal etc.

Home Postural Drainage

Patients may be taught home postural drainage so that they can perform the PD independently. Home PD can be performed by either using the pillows, newspaper etc. place a 15 cm (6 inch) pile of newspaper or magazines tied tightly together, in the centre of bed and place pillows on the top. The patient can lie over this in various positions to drain several areas of the lung. Sleeping in a couch with foot end propped up with bricks in the night is a method used to drain lower lobes. Alternate side lying is most commonly used position for patients with generalised secretions. Bending forward over the toilet, or leaning over to clean the bath, which are positions reported by some patients to spontaneously clear secretions. Babies and small children can be given postural drainage over their mother's knee. It is usually advisable to give the treatment before a feed.

Chapter 13

External Manipulations on Thorax or Chest Manipulations

Chest manipulations include:

- Percussion.
- Vibrations.
- Shaking.

Percussion

SYNONYM

Percussion is also referred to as cupping, clapping and tapotement.

DEFINITION

Percussion is an airway clearance technique that involves clapping on the chest and/or back to help loosen thick secretions. The purpose of percussion is to intermittently apply kinetic energy to the chest wall and lung. This is accomplished by rhythmically striking the thorax with cupped hand or mechanical device directly over the lung segment(s) being drained. Trapping the air between the patients thorax and the care givers hand dislodge or loosen bronchial secretions from airways so that they may be removed by suctioning or expectoration. The aim is to loosen the secretions, increases mucociliary transport. It is performed during both inspiratory and expiratory phases of breathing. It is used along with postural drainage and with ACBT technique.

Indications

Sputum volume or consistency suggesting a need for additional manipulation (e.g., percussion and/ or vibration) to assist movement of secretions by gravity, in a patient receiving postural drainage.

Equipments Required

1. *For adult people*
   A. **Manual**
      - Physiotherapist cupped hands or caregivers cupped hands.

   B. **Mechanical**
      - Electrical or pneumatic Percussors.

2. *For Infants*
   A. **Manual**
      - Four fingers cupped.
      - Three fingers with middle finger tented.
      - Thenar or hypothenar surfaces of hand.

   B. **Mechanical**
      - Padded rubber nipples.
      - Paediatric anesthesia masks.
      - Padded medicine cups.
      - Bell end of stethoscope.

Preparation

- PD positions.
- Place a thin towel.
- Adjust level of bed-body mechanics.

Technique

- Cupping with fingers, thumb adducted.
- Sound: Hollow sound than slapping sound.
- Rhythm: 100 to 480 times per minute.
- Start with non dominant followed by dominant.
- Percussion over bony prominence (spine of vertebrae, scapula, clavicle, floating ribs), breast should be avoided

Contraindications

- Subcutaneous emphysema.
- Recent epidural spinal infusion or spinal anesthesia.
- Recent skin grafts, or flaps, on the thorax.
- Burns, open wounds, and skin infections of the thorax.
- Recently placed transvenous pacemaker or subcutaneous pacemaker (particularly if mechanical devices are to be used).
- Suspected pulmonary tuberculosis.
- Lung contusion.
- Bronchospasm.
- Osteomyelitis of the ribs.
- Osteoporosis.
- Coagulopathy.
- Complaint of chest-wall pain.
- Rib metastasis.

Advantages

- Enhance secretion clearance.
- Shorten the PD treatment session.
- Soothing and sedation for young babies.

Disadvantages

- Care giver is necessary.
- Fatigue to the care giver.
- Not tolerated by post operative patients.
- Fall in oxygen saturation.

Vibrations and Shaking

DEFINITION

Vibration involves the application of a fine tremorous action (manually performed by pressing in the direction that the ribs and soft tissue of the chest move during expiration) over the draining area. Shaking is a stronger bouncing maneuver which supplies concurrent compressive force to chest wall. Vibrations are gentle high frequency force whereas shaking is more vigorous in nature. The aim is to move secretions from lung periphery to larger airways. Vibration is performed by co contraction of care givers upper limbs to cause vibrations while applying pressure to chest wall with the hands. Shaking and vibrations are performed only during expiratory phase.

Indications

Sputum volume or consistency suggesting a need for additional manipulation (e.g., percussion and/or vibration) to assist movement of secretions by gravity, in a patient receiving postural drainage.

Equipment Required

1. *Adults*

A. **Manual:** Caregiver or physiotherapist hand.

B. **Mechanical:** Vibrators.

2. *Infants*

A. **Manual:** With thumb and index finger or index with middle finger.

B. **Mechanical:** Padded electric tooth brush.

Preparation

- PD position.
- Thin towel.
- Adjust the level of bed–Body mechanics.

Procedure

A. *Frequency*

- **Vibrations:** 12-20 Hz.
- **Shaking:** 2 Hz.

B. *Placing*

- **For vibrations:** Hands may be placed side by side or on top of another. At the peak of inspiration apply vibration follow till chest wall deflation.
- **For shaking:** Place the hands over the lobe of the lungs. Instruct the patient to take deep breath. At the peak of inspiration apply a slow rhythmic bouncing pressure to chest wall until the end of expiration. The hand follow the movement of chest as the air is exhaled.

Contraindications

- Subcutaneous emphysema.
- Recent epidural spinal infusion or spinal anesthesia.
- Recent skin grafts, or flaps, on the thorax.
- Burns, open wounds, and skin infections of the thorax.
- Recently placed transvenous pacemaker or subcutaneous pacemaker (particularly if mechanical devices are to be used).
- Suspected pulmonary tuberculosis.
- Lung contusion.
- Bronchospasm.
- Osteomyelitis of the ribs.
- Osteoporosis.
- Coagulopathy.
- Complaint of chest-wall pain.
- Rib metastasis.

Advantages

- Enhance mobilization of secretions.
- Better tolerated than percussion.
- Encourage a deeper expiration to follow.

Disadvantage

- Can be applied only with care giver or therapist.

Chapter 14

Suctioning

DEFINITION

The suctioning can be defined as bronchohygenic technique which involves mechanical aspiration of pulmonary secretions by means of negative pressure application.

Indications

1. Need to remove secretions
   a. Whenever the secretions can be heard in an intubated patient (Noisy breaths).
   b. On auscultation with coarse breath sounds.
   c. If the inflation pressure (Peak Inspiratory Pressure) of ventilator suddenly rises, there may be large plug of mucus in one large bronchi or even within endotracheal or tracheostomy tube.
   d. If minute volume drops which indicate retained secretions.
   e. Changes in graphics, ABG's.
   f. Decreased tidal volume.
2. For retained secretions in spontaneously breathing patient who is unable to cough and expectorate or may be unwilling to cough or unable to cough due to confusion, pain, fear or in an unconscious patients or if respiratory muscles are paralyzed by disease or drugs.
3. Before and during the release of cuff on tracheostomy tube.
4. Need to obtain sputum specimen.
5. Need to stimulate cough.
6. Presence of atelectasis due to a large mucous plug.

Types of Suction

The types of suctioning are open and closed suction system. In an open suctioning patient ventilator is disconnected and suctioning is performed (Figure 14.1). In closed suction a multi-use suction catheter

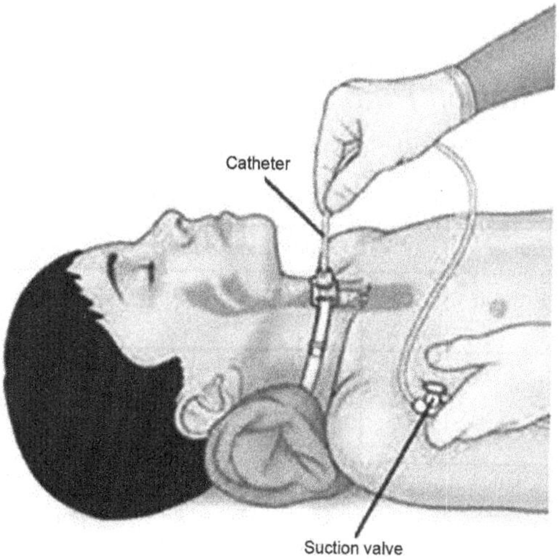

Fig. 14.1: Open suctioning system

are incorporated directly into the ventilator circuit and used repeatedly over 24 to 48 hours (Figure 14.2). Since suctioning can be performed without disconnecting the patient from the ventilator, high

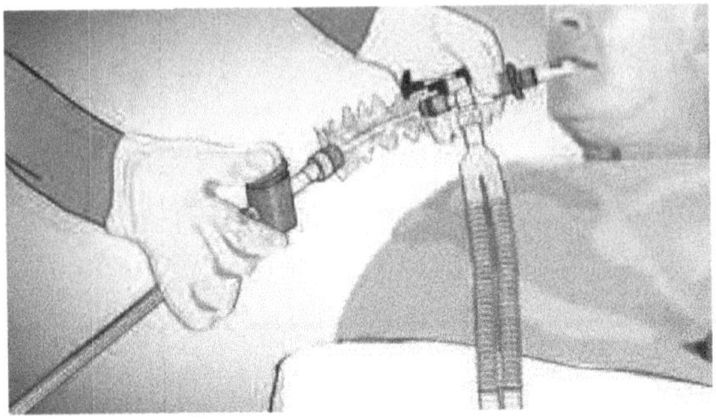

Fig. 14.2: Closed suctioning system

FiO_2 and PEEP can be maintained, resulting in less likelihood of hypoxemia (pre-oxygenation with 100% O_2 is still required). In addition, cross-contamination is less likely than with single-use catheters. However, the extra weight an in-line catheter adds to a ventilator circuit may increase tension on the tracheal tube. Also, the presence of the catheter in the airway increases resistance and can alter the volumes delivered by the ventilator. Last, the reduced airway pressure during suctioning can cause the ventilator to inadvertently trigger on. Comparison is given in Table 14.1.

Suction Equipment

1. *Suction Pumps*

A. Central Suction Apparatus

Parts: A vaccum point close to patients bed power is provided by large motor (which is far away from the patient) which an on/off switch, control dial which allows applied negative pressure to be increased or decreased, manometer, suction jar, connector, suction tubing and catheter (Figures 14.3 and 14.4).

Displays Pressure Settings

Low pressure: 50 mm of Hg.

Medium: 100 mm of Hg.

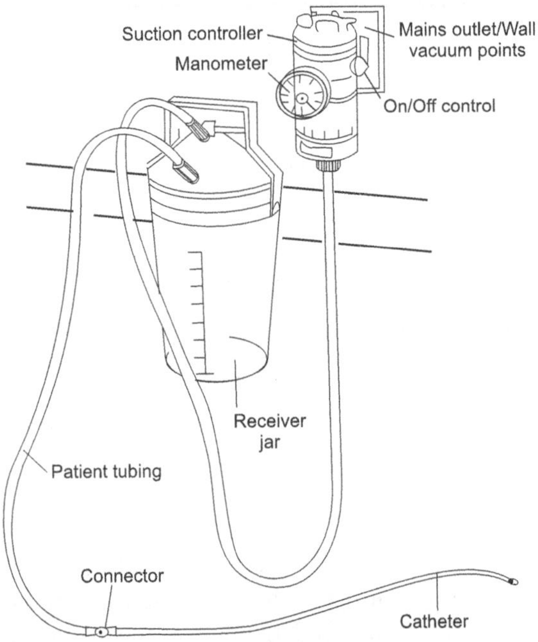

Fig. 14.3: Parts of central suction apparatus

Table 14.1 Comparison of open suction with closed suctioning

Features	*Open suctioning*	*Closed suctioning*
Definition	Patient ventilator system opened for suctioning	Patient ventilator system closed for suctioning
Advantages	Cheap Procedure not complicated	No infection No hypoxemia Reusable
Disadvantages	Infection Hypoxemia Single use of catheter	Expensive Complicated procedure Automatic triggering

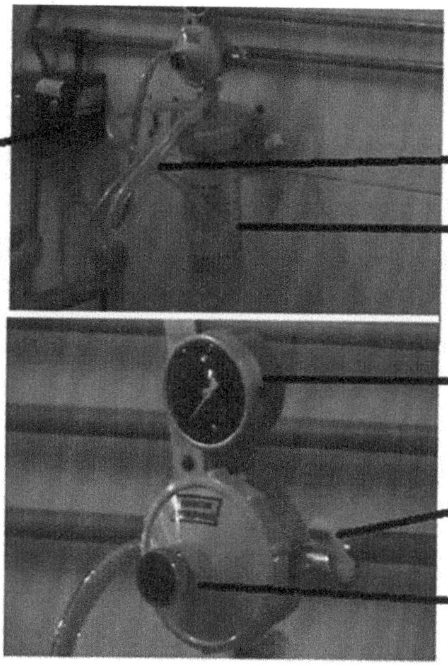

Fig. 14.4: Parts of central suction apparatus (See colour plate no. II)

High: 300 mm of Hg.

Recommended pressure settings are given in Table 14.2.

Table 14.2

Patient	*Recommended pressure*
Adult	-100 to -120 mm of Hg
Child	-80 to -100 mm of Hg
Infant	-60 to -80 mm of Hg

B. **Electrical Suction Apparatus:** Powered from mains, small motor, on/off switch, a control dial.

C. **Portable Suction Apparatus:** Powered by rechargeable batteries, small motor/on/off switch.

D. **Foot Pump:** Power is provided by operator. Used in the community or for an emergency resuscitation team.

2. Suction Bottle

All suction pumps have one bottle but electrically operated pumps have two.

3. Suction Tubing (Vacuum Tubing)

Connecting from suction bottle to suction catheter tubing is made from clear plastic for easy viewing.

4. Connections

It may be a Y connector (Figure 14.5B) or ribbed connector (Figure 14.5A). In case of ribbed connector one end connects to vaccum tubing and other end connects to the suction catheter. The end which connects catheter has thumb control valve. In the case of Y connector, three arms. One at either end and third at the side used as control port some have inbuilt control ports. To apply suction force to catheter operator places thumb over opening.

5. Catheters

Catheters used for open suctioning:

A. **Plastic, Sterile, Non-disposable:** It should not exceed half the diameter of endotracheal or tracheotomy tube. Too large catheter may

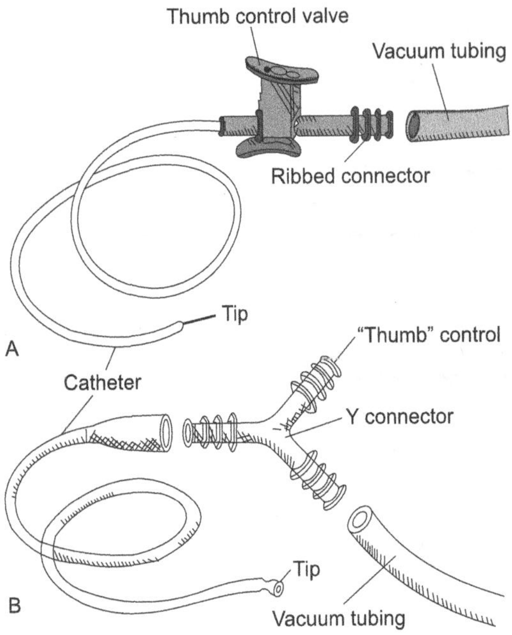

Fig. 14.5: Connector

cause alveolar collapse. The distal tip of catheters may be either 90 degree cut or 45 degree cut. Delee catheters have the distal tip cut at a 90 degree angle. Whistle tip catheters are cut at a 45 degree angle (See Figure 14.6).

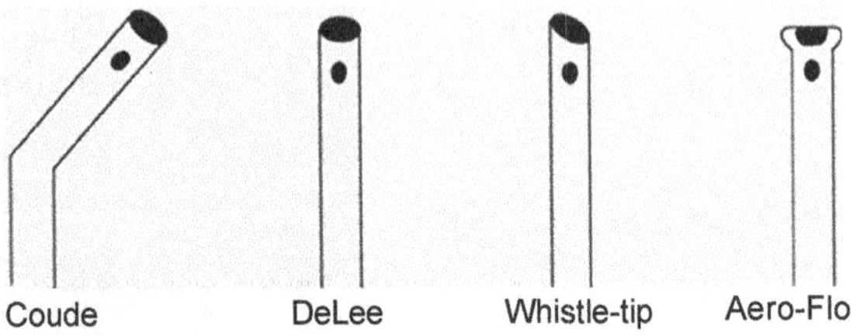

Fig. 14.6: Suction catheters

Suction catheter is detailed in Figure 14.7A. Each catheter is color coded. It can be of plain, thumb control, T type or finger tip control (Figure 14.7B). In French Gauge (FG) starting from the smallest size of 5 FG to the largest size of 24 FG (Figure 14.7B).

Size in FG	Colour	Plain	Thumb Control	Finger Tip Control
5	Grey			
6	Light Green			
8	Blue			
10	Black			
12	White			
14	Green			
16	Orange			
18	Red			
20	Yellow			
22	Violet			
24	Light Blue			

Fig. 14.7A: Suction catheter of different size with color code (See colour plate no. II)

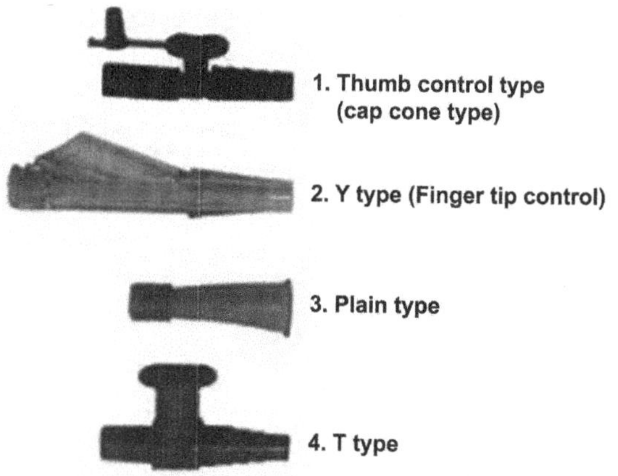

Fig. 14.7B (See colour plate no. III)

B. **Soft rubber catheter** is still used in some hospitals. These are not disposable and must be sterilized after use, cause less trauma because they are softer and more flexible than plastic catheters. They may be too short for some endotracheal tubes.

C. **Coudes catheter** (also Bronchitrac), is a long catheter with a curved tip used for suctioning left main bronchus. Head side should flex to right side (See Figure 14.6).

D. **Aeroflo Catheters:** Those undergone laryngeal or tracheal surgery or patients undergoing anticoagulation therapy even minimal trauma would be dangerous. These catheters have a bead surrounding the distal hole at the end of catheter. There are four small holes just proximal to this bead (See Figure 14.6).

E. **Sputum trap** may be used when bronchial secretion needs to be sent for laboratory investigations.

F. **Dual Catheters:** The Jinotti O_2 insufflation catheter has a dual-lumen so O_2 can be delivered while suctioning.

Catheters used for closed suctioning:

These are continuous use suction (catheters reused upto 24-48 hours). The catheter is covered with a sleeve (*See* Figure 14.8).

6. Suction Trolley

It contains sterile plastic gloves, catheters, lubricating jelly (water based) for nasopharyngeal, Sterile gauze swabs to transfer jelly to tip of catheter, Bowl of sodium bicarbonate or sterile water for flushing, Plastic bag for collection of disposables, Bowl of antiseptics for collection of items to be sterilized.

Mode of Entry

1. Nasopharyngeal

- Patients' neck is extended.
- Catheter advanced on inspiration.
- Very unpleasant experience.
- This entry should not be used with head injuries with CSF leaks into passages.

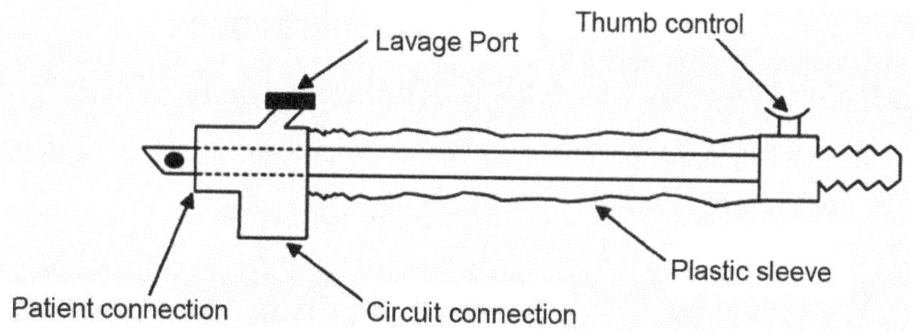

Fig. 14.8: Continuous use of suction catheter

2. *Oropharyngeal.*

3. *Suction via Tube*

a. Endotracheal.
b. Tracheostomy.
c. Minitracheostomy.

Prior to Suctioning

- Adjust FiO_2 on mechanical ventilation.
- Temporary oxygen enrichment.
- Manual ventilation.
- Use of dual catheter.
- Sigh breaths.

Precautions During Suctioning

1. No suction pressure is applied while catheter is being introduced. Airway suctioning causes mucosal trauma.
2. Catheter should be advanced until either a cough reflex is elicited or some resistance in the trachea is encountered.
3. Gentle rolling of the catheter between the finger and the thumb ensures continuous rotation to minimize the tracheal trauma.
4. Interrupted suction should always be used to prevent build up of the negative pressure.
5. If the pool of secretion is reached there may be a pause to clear them. While continuing to rotate the catheter.
6. Vigorous up and down movement (Thrombo-ning method) is not used.
7. Observe the patient of the signs of hypoxia.
8. If during the nasopharyngeal suction patient becomes cyanosed and the catheter is difficult to remove then disconnect the suction leaving the catheter *in situ*.
9. No longer than 15 sec should elapse between the disconnection and reconnection of the patient to the ventilator.
10. Whenever possible patient should be suctioned inside lying with head rotated to one side to avoid the aspiration of the gastric contents.
11. All equipments and supplies should be properly disposed off.

Hazards

1. *Risk of infection patient or care giver*

Prevented by good sterile technique.

2. *Trauma*

Prevented by correct choice of catheter and control negative pressure by good technique.

3. *Hypoxia*

Prevented by accurate use of applied negative pressure and accurate timing.

4. *Cardiac arrhythmia*

Prevented by breathing higher concentration of O_2 prior to suctioning.

5. *Atelectasis*

Prevented by use of dual catheters or closed suction system.

Complications

Bronchospasm

Due to presence of any foreign body.

Elevated ICP

An increase in ICP during suctioning is usually due to arterial hypertension or coughing.

Hypertension/Hypotension

- Hypotension during suctioning may be due to cardiac arrhythmias or severe coughing episodes that decrease venous return.
- Hypertension may be caused by hypoxemia or increased sympathetic tone due to stress, anxiety, pain, or change in hemodynamics resulting from manual hyperventilation.

Interruption of Mechanical Ventilation

During suctioning time, the mechanical ventilation is interrupted and PEEP is lost which results in significant hypoxemia.

Cardiorespiratory Arrest

Cardiac arrhythmia due to suctioning procedure may sometime leads to cardiorespiratory arrest.

Note: Suctioning procedure may result in tachycardia or bradycardia. Hypoxemia due to suctioning can result in tachycardia. An awake patient may become anxious by seeing the suctioning procedure which also results in tachycardia. If a catheter tip touches the carina, vagal receptors are stimulated and may result in bradycardia.

Use the following formula to estimate the maximum French size suction catheter for the ID of an endotracheal or tracheostomy tube:

Maximum diameter (Fr) of catheter = ID of endotracheal tube*3/2.

For example to calculate the largest suction catheter that should be used with a size 8 (ID) endotracheal tube:

$$8*3/2 = 24/2=12 \text{ FG}$$

Therefore, a 12 Fr suction catheter could be used with an 8 mm ID endotracheal (or tracheostomy) tube.

Knowing the ID of a suction catheter is helpful because it relates to the maximum particle size that can pass through it. The following formula can be used to interconvert from French OD to millimeters ID:

$$\text{mm} = (\text{Fr}-2)/4$$

What is the ID in millimeters of a 12 Fr suction catheter?

$$\text{mm} = 2.5$$

$$\text{mm} = 12-2/4$$

$$= 10/4$$

$$2.5$$

Therefore, a 12 Fr suction catheter (with a 4 mm OD) can be used to suction particles up to 2.5 mm in diameter.

Chapter 15

Autogenic Drainage

HISTORY

Jean Chevalier in Belgium in 1967.

Kraimar *ét al.* modified in 1986.

DEFINITION

This technique is method of controlled breathing in which patient adjust the rate, location and depth of respiration.

Rationale

Postural drainage which is given for young asthmatics to bring out secretions produce harm rather than bringing out secretions. Hence autogenic drainage is preferred than PD in these patients.

Aims

- To improve clearance of mucus.
- To improve ventilation.
- To maintain optimal chest wall movement.

Methods

- Belgian Approach.
- German Approach.

Belgian Approach

At the beginning of this breathing technique inspiration is performed slowly through nose to provide optimal humidification and warming of inspired air. This help to prevent coughing (Figure 15.1).

1. **Peripheral Loosening of Mucus (unsticky phase)**

   This phase is directed at increased inspiration is followed by deep expiration, and then the mid tidal volume is lowered in range of normal expiratory reserve volume.

   Secretions from peripheral lung regions are mobilised by compression of peripheral alveolar duct.

2. **Collection of Mucus in Larger Airways (collecting phase)**

   In this phase tidal volume breathing is then changed gradually from expiratory reserve volume to inspiratory reserve volume to mobilise secretions from apical regions. Longer the expiration time greater the distance that secretion will be transported.

3. **Transport of mucus from larger airways to mouth (evacuating phase)**

   In this phase patient increases respiratory flow starting from the level at about the middle of

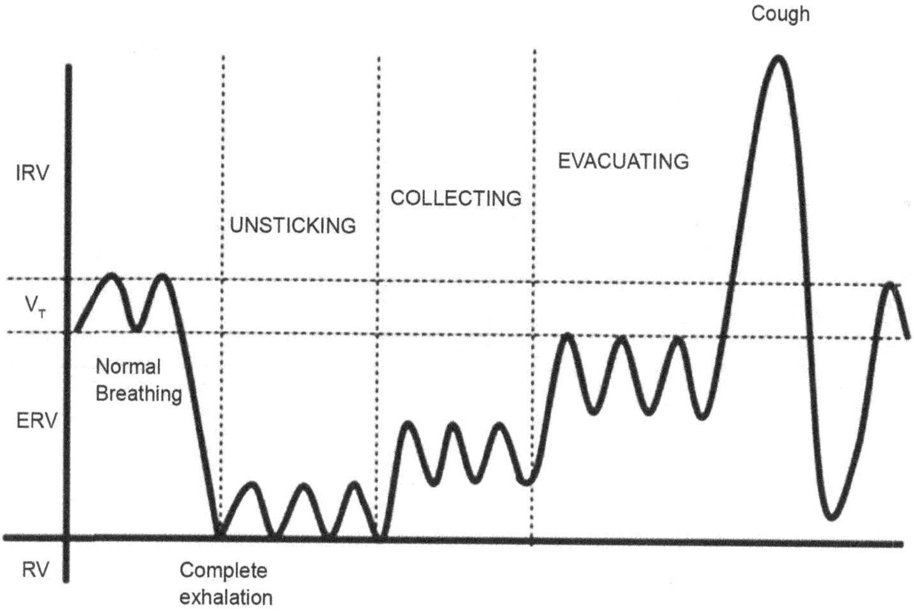

Fig. 15.1: Phases of autogenic drainage

inspiratory reserve capacity added by short burst of very gentle coughing. Autogenic drainage performed twice a day patient seated in firm upright position usually performed after inhalation of nebulised drugs.

German Approach

In this approach it is not split into three phases. Rationale is such that respiration in expiratory reserve volume range seldom took place because patients were uncomfortable when breathing at low mid tidal volume and expiration is forbidden in second phase even if the patient clearly ready to do so.

Advantages

- Patients can perform independently by patients over 12 years of age.
- It does not require an additional equipment.
- It does not require use of PD positions hence it is appropriate for patients with GER.
- It is also recommended for use in patients with airway hyper reactivity.

Disadvantages

- Patient who is unmotivated or uncooperative.
- Children under 4 years of age.

Chapter 16

Active Cycle Breathing Technique (ACBT)

HISTORY

Thompson (1973): Combined forced expirations and diaphragmatic breathing.

FET (1979): Forced expiration technique.

ACBT (1993): ACBT consists of three phases: Breathing Control, Thoracic expansion and FET.

Components of Phases

Breathing Control Phase

Gentle tidal volume breathing with relaxation of upper chest and shoulders.

Thoracic Expansion Phase

Consist of deep inspiration and accompanied by percussion, vibration, usually given by care givers. This helps to loosen secretions.

Forced Expiratory Technique (FET)

This involves one and two huffs (forced expirations) from mid-lung volume and continued down to low lung volume will move secretions from peripheral to upper airway. Upper airway secretions are cleared by huff from high lung volume.

Significance of the Phases

Breathing Control

To prevent bronchospasm.

Thoracic Expansion

To increase lung volume, promotes collateral ventilation allowing air to get behind secretions assist in their mobilisation.

FET

It is based on "equal pressure point theory" by Mead *et al.*

It is the point in the airways where airway pressure is equal to pleural pressure. FET produces compression of airways peripherally to EPP. A huff from high lung volume causes compression within the trachea and bronchi to move secretions from these larger airways.

Position

A sitting or postural drainage position can be adopted. A minimum of 10 minutes in any productive position may be necessary to clear a patient.

Effects

- Because huffing has been shown to stabilise collapsible bronchial walls, it increases expiratory flow in the patients with obstruction without causing airway collapse.
- Decrease in oxygen saturation has been demonstrated with postural drainage and percussion has been prevented with use of ACB technique.

Equipment Required

For percussion, shaking and vibration on the chest wall during thoracic expansion patient or care givers hands can be used otherwise mechanical percussors or vibrators can be used. If PD positions are used equipment for positioning such as tilt table or pillows will be required. To teach huffing maneuver in infants a Peak flow meter mouthpiece can be used to blow of small cotton balls which is called as game of huffing at the cotton balls. According to Mahl Meister, 1991 a 'Chicken breath' can be adopted for children. In this method children are asked to adduct shoulder rapidly which comes and tap the lateral side of the thorax. This resembles a percussion which aids in the clearance of secretions. This is administered in phase of thoracic expansion.

PROCEDURE

Breathing Control

The patient is instructed to breath in a relaxed manner using normal tidal volume. The upper chest and shoulder remains relaxed and lower chest and abdomen should be active. The phase of breathing control should last as long as patients require relaxation and preparation for next phases usually 5 to 10 seconds. The breathing control resembles diaphragmatic breathing with the exception that in breathing control patients are instructed to do a normal tidal volume breath.

Thoracic Expansion

This phase emphasises on inspiration. Patients are instructed to take deep breath into inspiratory reserve volume and expiration is passive and relaxed. Chest percussion, shaking vibration may be performed in combination with thoracic expansion as patient exhale.

FET Technique

Forced expiratory technique is a forced expiration or huff combined with periods of breathing control one or two huffs from mid lung volume to low lung volume in which peripheral secretions are mobilised. Two different levels of huffing are used in this phase. A huff after medium sized breath will be effective to mobilise secretions from peripheral airways. This huff will be longer and quieter. Huff after deep breath will be effective to clear secretions that have reached the larger proximal airways. One or two huffs or cough at high lung volume will clear secretions from upper airways. This will be shorter and larger. After one or two huffs, patient must pause for breathing control to prevent bronchospasm (Figure 16.1).

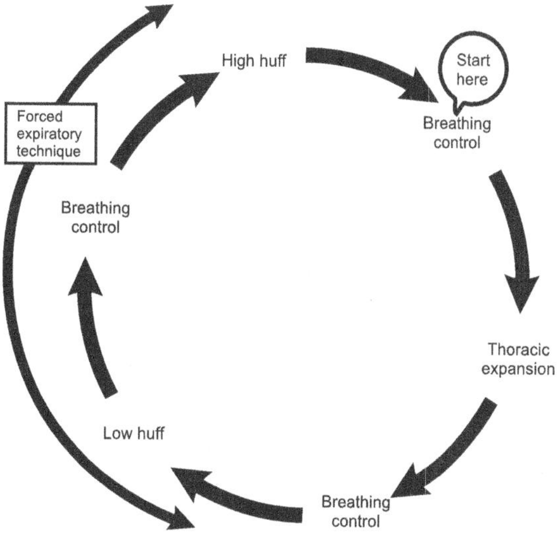

Fig. 16.1: Sequence of ACBT

Termination of Exercise

When a huff from medium sized inspiration through complete expiration is non-productive and dry sounding for two cycles in a row the treatment may be concluded.

Advantages

- Patient can actively participate in secretion mobilisation.
- Independently managing airway clearance.
- Technique may be adapted for patients with gastroesophagial reflex, bronchospasm and acute exacerbation of pulmonary disease.
- Decrease in oxygen saturation caused by chest percussion can be avoided by ACBT.
- Cost of ACBT is minimal.

Disadvantages

- In young children and extremely ill adults a care giver will be necessary to assist the patient this technique.
- Care must be taken to adapt technique in patient with hyperactive airways.

Chapter 17

Other Airway Clearance Techniques

Turning

Turning is the rotation of the body around the longitudinal axis. Turning is also referred to as kinetic therapy or continuous lateral rotational therapy. Less aggressive forms of turning include various rotational therapies such as kinetic therapy, in which patients are rotated from side to side in a turn of at least 40°, and continuous lateral rotation therapy (CLRT), in which patients are rotated from side to side in a turn of less than 40°. Patients may turn themselves or be turned by a caregiver or use a special rotational bed. Special rotational beds, such as the Roto-Rest Bed (Kinetic Concepts, Inc. San Antonio, Texas) rotate continuously on their long axis through a 124-degree arc every 3 to 4 minutes (encompassing kinetic therapy and CLRT). This bed allowed continuous turning up to 62° (124° arc).

Role of Exercise in Airway Clearance

Exercise increases transpulmonary pressure gradient, increases mucociliary transport, boosts collateral ventilation thereby opening closed bronchi, increases expiratory flow. Exercise leads to sympathetic stimulation of cilia by catecholamine release and parasympathetic stimulation of airway mucous glands. Exercise induces cough thereby clearing secretions. Aerobic exercise is preferred for secretion clearance. Exercise can be done with treadmill, bicycle ergometer, elliptical trainer, mini trampoline or arm ergometer. Exercise is not suitable for very young children less than 5 years of age, patients with neuromascular weakness and those who are with acute exacerbation of COPD or asthma.

Cornet

Positive pressures and oscillations can be created by actively breathing out through a curved plastic tube called a cornet. This contains a flexible hose, which acts as a valve. Studies have shown that it decreases sputum viscosity.

High Frequency Chest Wall Oscillation (HFCWO) or High Frequency Chest Compression (HFCC)

It consists of an inflatable vest linked to an air pulse generator. This provides oscillations of thoracic cavity between 5-25 Hz. The lung volume expired tends to increase with lower frequency (< 10 Hz) whereas the flow rates tends to increase with higher frequency (>10 Hz). The working principle of HFCWO is by differential air flow. The expiratory flow rate is higher than the inspiratory flow rate. This allows the mucous to transport from periphery to central airways. The oscillatory airflow leads to changes in consistency of mucous. The difference between the expiratory and inspiratory velocities produces shear forces strong enough to move mucous.

Intrapulmonary Percussive Ventilation (IPPV)

IPPV simultaneously delivers intrathoracic percussion and aerosolized solution for bronchodilation. The apparatus known as the phasitron is the main component of this ventilator. This provides high frequency impulses during inspiration, while positive expiratory pressure is maintained throughout passive exhalation. The pressure is generated is between 10 and 30 cm of H_2O. Compared to HFCC which delivers oscillation externally, IPPV delivers internally. The changes in the frequency and pressure of the airflow delivered through the IPPV device assist in stabilizing the airways and decrease the viscosity of the secretions. This mobilizes secretions.

Frequencer

The frequencer is a device that provides mechanical vibration in addition to acoustic oscillation to mobilise secretions through a variety of tissue depths. The frequencer operates between 20 and 65 Hz. The device adjusts to the resonant frequency of the airways of the lungs and is able to target small portions of the lungs. The mechanism is same as that of the HFCWO.

Mechanical In-Exsufflation or Cough Assist Machine

In this type of bronchial hygiene therapy both positive pressures and negative pressures are used. This device allows gradual application of positive pressure which is quickly shifted to a negative pressure. Rapid change in pressure produces high expiratory flow rate stimulating a cough. This assists in removal of secretions and normalisation of SPO_2.

Table 17.1: Advantages and disadvantages of airway clearance techniques

Device	*Advantages*	*Disadvantages*
Exercise	Only technique performed regularly Care giver support is not required Equipments not required as simple walking is enough No cost	Patient may not tolerate the frequency of exercise Cannot be given during acute exacerbation Cannot be given with neurological and musculoskeletal limitations Patients adherence may be lost to the program
Postural drainage	Easy to learn Can be coordinated with other bed care activities Cost is minimal Home PD can be coordinated with activities such as reading or watching television	Optimal PD positions are contraindicated Children may not adhere to the program
Percussion	Can shorten the time of PD position if it is added For young children it is rhythm soothing, relaxed and often sedated	Not tolerated by post-operative patients Contraindicated in coagulative and osteoporotic patients

Contd.

Contd.

Vibrations and shaking	Better tolerated than percussion Suitable for post-operative patients Simultaneously pattern and depth can be assessed	Care givers assistance is required Contraindicated in coagulative and osteoporotic patients
High frequency chest wall oscillation	Suitable for young children (> 2 years) Also for large and obese adults For patients whom PD is contraindicated Patients who cannot tolerate upright position Time saving Contact time of patient with caregiver is less	High cost Lack of portability
Intrapulmonary percussive ventilation	Used for home use and hospital Independent use Less expensive than HFCWO	Not tolerated by young children Less literature support
Acoustic airway clearance (Frequencer)	Do not required to alter the breathing pattern Treatment can be focused to specific areas in the lung Nebulized medication or supplemental oxygen can be given simultaneously	High cost Less literature support
Kinetic therapy	Can reduce ventilator associated pneumonia Prevent atelectasis	High cost Patient has to be sedated to improve tolerance of bed rotation
Mechanical in-exsufflation	Useful in neuromascular disorders Used in weaning	Sudden bradycardia or tachycardia Can produce gastroesophageal reflux with aspiration Produce nausea

Chapter 18

Manual Hyperinflation

HISTORY

First described by Clement and Hubsch in 1968.

DEFINITION

Delivering the gas to the patient with an inflating bag can be achieved by three ways and they are defined below:

A. Manual Hyperinflation

- Inflating the lung with oxygen and manual compression to total volume (V_T) of liter requiring a peak inspiratory pressure of between 20 and 40 cmH_2O. (*Windsor et al.,1972*).
- Providing a larger tidal volume (V_T) than base line V_T to the patient and using a V_T, which is 50% greater than that delivered by the ventilator (*Singer et al., 1994*).

B. Manual Ventilation

- Squeezing gas into the patient's lungs at a normal tidal volume. For e.g., when changing ventilator tubing, or transfer of patient from ICU to ward or Investigation room.

C. Manual Hyperventilation

- Delivering rapid breaths more than normal breath. For e.g., if patient is hypercapnic. Manual hyperventilation reduces $PaCO_2$ which results in vasoconstriction thereby reducing brain oedema and ICP.

Indications

- To help clinical assessment of air entry into lungs.
- To improve oxygenation pre and post suctioning.
- To mobilize excess bronchial secretion.
- To re-inflate areas of collapsed lungs.
- To maintain ventilation when mechanical is interrupted.

TYPES OF DELIVERY

Air can be delivered through Mapleson circuit or through self-inflating bag.

A. Mapleson Circuit

Mapleson circuit is characterised by absence of valves to direct from or to the patient. But when inspiratory gas flow exceeds fresh gas flow rebreathing occurs. Its components include Reservoir bag, corrugated tubing, Adjustable pressure limiting valve, Fresh gas inlet, patient connection (Figure 18.1). Based on their relative position it is classified into 6 different types (Figure 18.2). Normally it is used in anesthesia breathing systems. It can be also used as manual hyperinflation and used in many parts of the world.

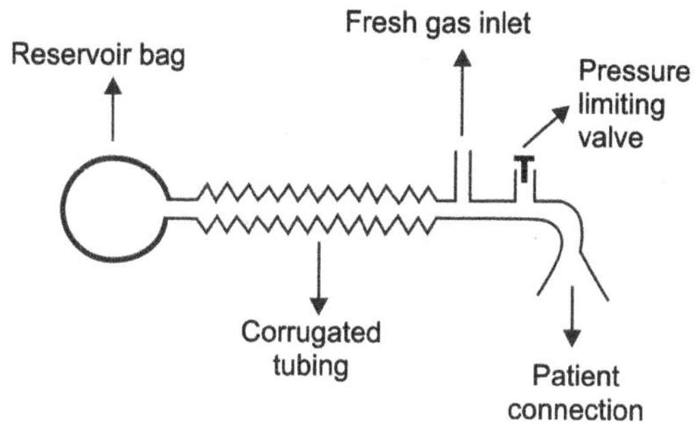

Fig. 18.1: Parts of Mapleson circuit

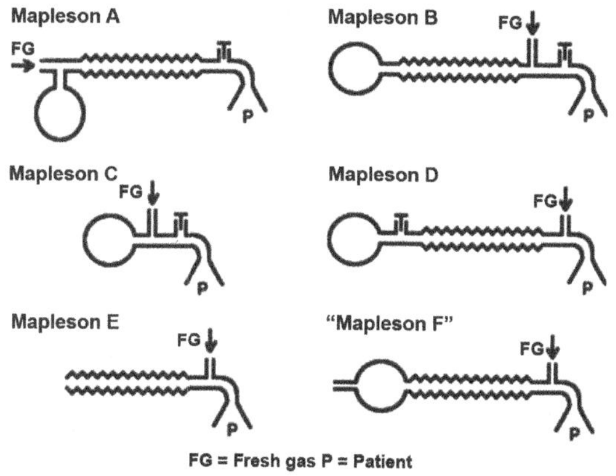

Fig. 18.2: Classification of Mapleson circuit

B. Self Inflating Bag

Self-inflating bag has inbuilt valve that's prevent rebreathing. Bag should be more compliant to feel compliance of lungs. Two types of self-inflating bags are commercially available; Laerdal bag and Air Viva bag. A study showed that PEFR was highest in Laerdal bag followed by Air Viva and finally by Mapleson.

AMBU bag: It is a self-inflating bag (Figure 18.3). It is called as artificial manual Breathing unit. An AMBU bag can be used to re-expand the collapsed lungs. This can be achieved by slowing the inspiration and a hold is given at the end of inspiration. It can be also used for airway clearance therapy. This can be achieved by making faster expiration compared to inspiration. The parts of AMBU bag are patient adapter, Oxygen inlet, two Valves; Fish mouth valve (open during inspiration) and exhalation Valve (open during exhalation), Silicone bag (2 L for adults and 500 mL for pediatric), pressure limiting valve and Reservoir (Figure 18.4).

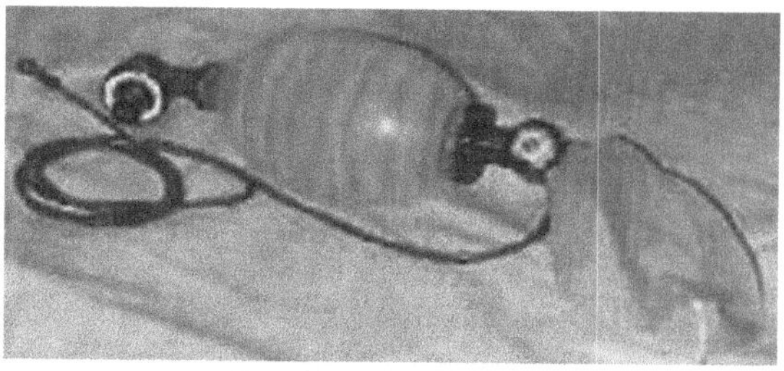

Fig. 18.3: An AMBU bag

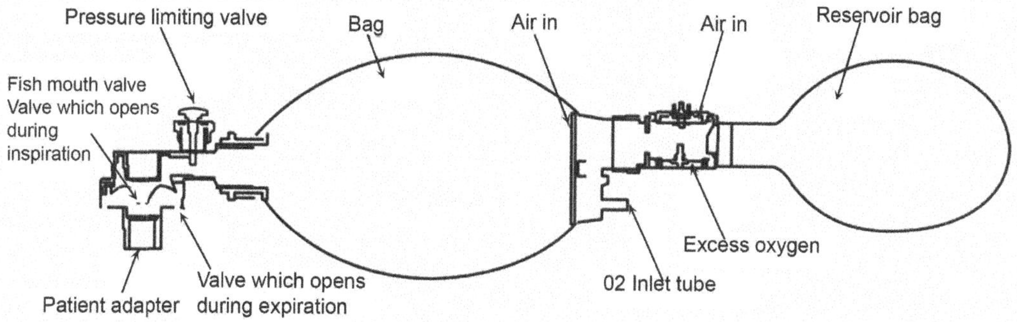

Fig. 18.4: Parts of AMBU bag

Feedback

Manual hyperinflation may increase the risk of trauma if high peak airway pressure and volumes are delivered. It should be more than 20 cm H_2O to be clinically effective and less than 40 cm H_2O to prevent barotrauma.

So to ensure safety there are subjective methods and objective methods.

A. **Subjective methods:** It can be analysed by following three ways:
   - Feeling the degree of tension in resuscitation bag.
   - Observing chest wall movement.
   - Listening to the air escaping through the valve.

   Disadvantage is that it is augmented by qualitative visual information about pressure being delivered. The order of compliance is in the following order; Mapleson > Air viva > Laerdal.

B. **Objective methods:** A pressure manometer can be connected in series with adapter. This gives the pressure reading. Adjust the pressure such that it should be more than 20 cm H_2O to be clinically effective and less than 40 cm H_2O.

Mechanism of Removal of Secretion:

Movement of secretion is by two-phase gas liquid transport. Gas flowing across a liquid imparts motion to liquid. Energy is transmitted from moving air to static liquid shearing and moving liquid in direction of the flow. This type of liquid flow can be bubble, slug, annular and mist according to the velocity. Faster velocity produces commonly annular and mist flow. Manual hyperinflation remove secretion by means of stimulating a cough but it did not produce expiratory flow rates of cough. High expiratory flow with dynamic change in airway diameter results in annular and mist flow (Figure 18.5). This results in expulsion of secretion. This is achieved by low I : E ratio. Ideal I : E ratio should be less than 0.9.

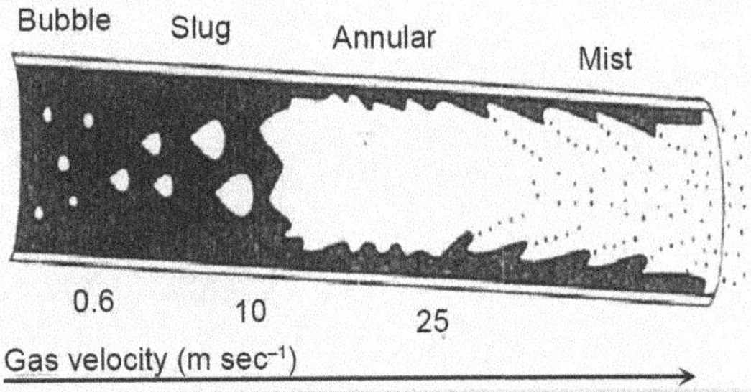

Fig. 18.5: Mechanism of removal of secretions

Factors that Influence I : E Ratio

- Diameter of endotracheal tube.
- Patient's pulmonary pathology.
- Operator performance (rate and amount of bag compression).
- Type of circuit, degree of valve closure.
- Low target volume.

Effects of Manual Hyperinflation

A. Beneficial Effects

- Increase static compliance.
- Increase removal of secretion.

B. Adverse Effects

- **Decrease cardiac output:** Increase intrathoracic volume causes decrease venous return by compression great veins, which results in reduction of cardiac output.
- **Increase intracranial pressure:** Increase intrathoracic volume causes decrease venous return, which causes increases stasis of blood in brain.

Precaution

- Fall in cardiac output.
- Barotraumas.
- Severe bronchospasm.

Contraindication

- Unstable cardiovascular system.
- Pneumothorax.
- Hypoxia.

Ventilator Sigh Mode Vs Manual Resuscitator

A study by Stone *et al.*, has shown that hyperinflation breaths delivered via ventilator are superior or equivalent to MRB in preventing suction induced hypoxemia. Delivery using MRB results in increased airway pressure and increased hemodynamic consequence. Clark *et al.* measured tidal volumes and inflation pressure generated during manual hyperinflation in ventilated patients and found that there is a negative correlation between average tidal volume and lung injury score. There was a positive correlation between peak inflation pressure and lung injury score.

Chapter 19

Hydration and Humidification

HYDRATION

Introduction

If a patient is well hydrated the secretions will be easily loosened up so it is better to advice the patient to drink warm water prior to chest physiotherapy.

Rationale

Dehydration reduces mucus transport by 25%.

Advantages

- Cheap.
- Safe.
- Not baffled out in the upper airways (Baffling discussed in chapter nebuliser).

Cause of Dehydration

- Stress incontinence due to chronic cough.
- Increased frequency due to diuretics.
- Change in environment and daily routine.
- Inability to reach their drink.
- Unwilling to bother busy staff.

HUMIDIFICATION

Definition

Method by which humidified (warming and moistening) air can be introduced into respiratory system.

Rationale

Normal humidification boundary is called as iso-thermic saturation boundary. It is 5 cm below carina but never below respiratory bronchioles. Humidification never happens beyond respiratory bronchioles. The natural humidification process reduces with reduced temperature, mouth breathers, with increased tidal volume or increased rate and with insertion of airways.

Indications

1. *Primary*
   (a) Humidifying dry medical gases.
   (b) Overcoming humidity deficit when upper airways is bypassed.
2. *Secondary*
   (a) Managing hypothermia.

(b) Treating bronchospasm caused by cold air.

Physical Principles Governing Humidifier Function

Temperature: More the temperature, more water vapor it can hold.

Surface Area: More surface area, more the humidification.

Contact Time: More contact time more the evaporation.

Classification

Classification 1: Boys and Howells Classification

1. **Suppliers**
   a. Vapor humidifier
      i. Ambient temperature vapor suppliers.
      ii. Heated vapor suppliers.
   b. Aerosol or nebulised humidifier
      i. Ambient temperature aerosol suppliers.
      ii. Heated aerosol suppliers.
2. **Conservers:** Heat moist exchanger (HME).

Classification 2 (Unnamed)

1. **Active**
   a. Low flow
      i. Bubble.
      ii. Passover.
   b. High flow
      i. Wick.
      ii. Cascade.
      iii. Vapor phase humidifier.
2. **Passive**
   a. Heat moist exchanger
      i. Hygroscopic.
      ii. Hydrophobic.

Types of Humidifier

Boys and Howells (1972) classified humidifiers into suppliers and conservers of water, and subdivided the former group.

Suppliers

Ambient Temperature Vapour Suppliers

Gas is bubbled through room temperature water; if passed through a very fine sieve so that the bubbles are very tiny then some useful humidification can perhaps be obtained.

Heated Vapour Suppliers

Gas is passed across or, preferably, through hot water or it may be dripped onto a very hot plate. The patient tubing may be lagged, or heated as in the Fischer-Paykell device, to prevent temperature loss and 'rain out'. It is vital that no danger of burning the patient exists, and these devices must not be capable of delivering gas at over 39°C to the patient end of the circuit; some of safety feedback cut-off mechanism from a thermometer close to the patient will probably become needed.

Ambient Aerosol Suppliers

These produce a mist of liquid water, either by breaking up water entrained by a high pressure gas jet (Bernoulli principle) or by generating the mist with a high speed spinning disc or an ultrasonic vibrating crystal. Ultrasonic nebulisation produces a very dense mist and there is a real danger of overloading the patient with water. A recently available device uses Babington principle, whereby air is forced through a fine film of water, and this produces a particularly dense mist.

Heated Aerosol Suppliers

The water to be nebulised is heated, and in particular the Bernoulli-type devices are often made to take a heating element or 'hot rod'. Thermal safety again is essential. Water may be simply added to the airway by direct instillation from a syringe, drip set or pump.

Conservers

These heat and moisture exchangers (HMEs), or condenser humidifiers, trap expired heat and water in a mesh, and return it to fresh inspired gas.

Bubble Through Humidifier (Analogous to Ambient Temperature Vapor Supplier)

Bubble through humidifier is used with nasal cannula, simple face mask and reservoir mask where the flow rate of dry oxygen is less. The smaller the bubbles, greater the content of the water in the delivered gas because of increased gas water interface. The factors which affect humidity in this humidifier are water level and the flow rate of the gas. If increased water column is provided there will be maximum water contact, so there will be more humidification. Higher the flow rate cools the water, decreasing its evaporative capacity and reducing contact time (Figure 19.1).

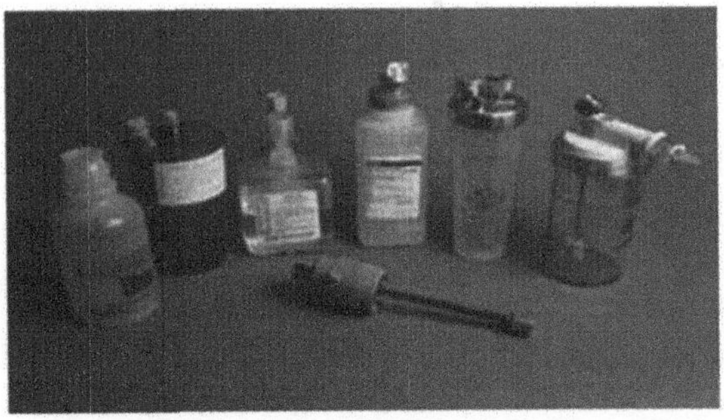

Fig. 19.1: Bubble through humidifier

Pass Over Humidifier

In this humidifier, gas passes over a heated water bath. Rising water vapor enters the gas, which is then transported to the patient (Figures 19.2 and 19.3).

Air entering and leaving shown in arrow marks.

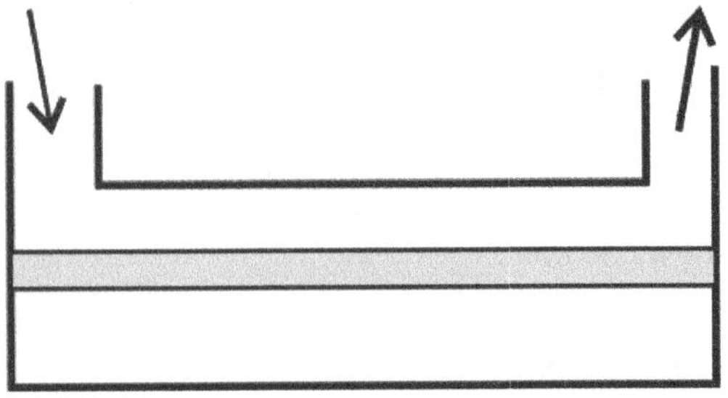

Fig. 19.2: Structure of passover humidifier

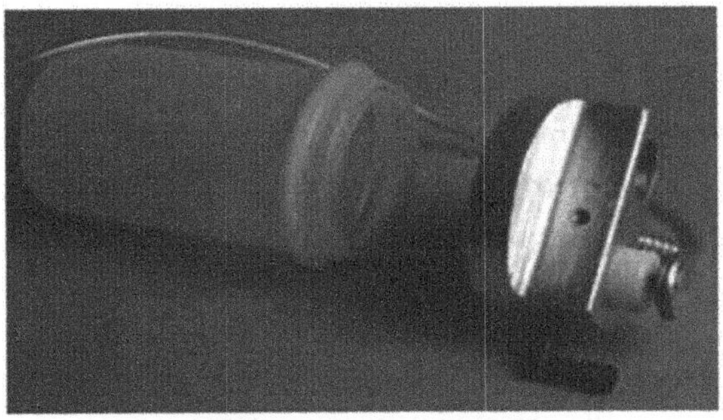

Fig. 19.3: A commercial type of passover humidifier

Wick Humidifier

In this humidifier, some material such as paper or composite material is partially submerged in the water. This material absorbs water and serves as the wick. Gases are humidified as they circulate around or through saturated wick (Figures 19.4 and 19.5).

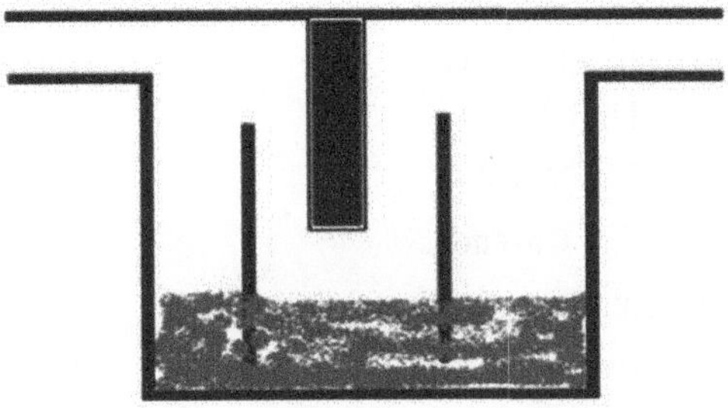

Fig. 19.4: Structure of wick humidifier

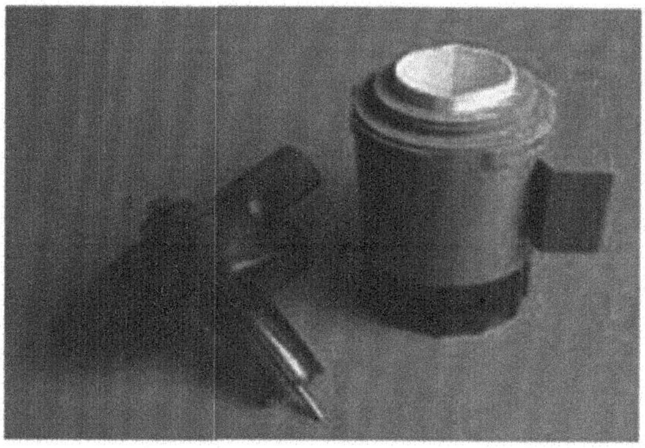

Fig. 19.5: A commercial type of wick humidifier

Cascade Humidifier

In this humidifier gas travels to the bottom of the cascade of water and is forced through a grid or mesh, creating fine bubbles. In addition gas flow emerges from under the water. Thus it is directed across the surface of the water. This increases the contact time and has the effect of increasing humidification. It can provide 100% humidity over a desired temperature (Figure 19.6).

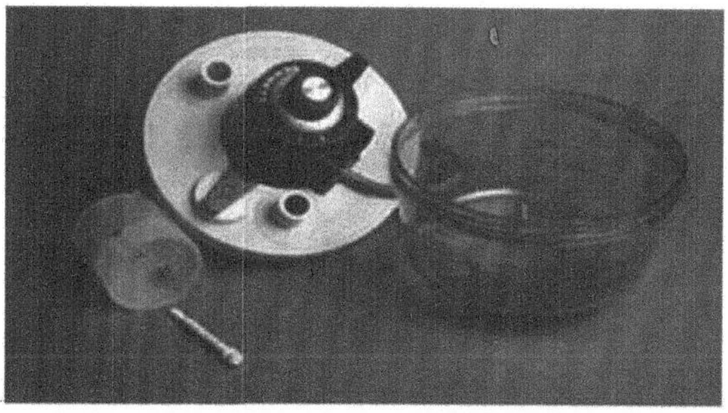

Fig. 19.6: A commercial type of cascade humidifier

Parts of heated humidifier for e.g., Fisher and Paykell humidifier (Figure 19.7).

- Heat source.
- Delivery tube.
- Temp monitor.
- Thermostat.
- Control.
- Alarms.

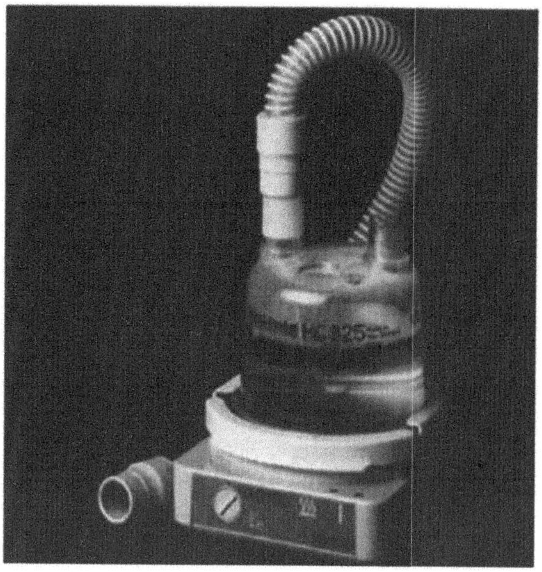

Fig. 19.7: Fisher and Paykell humidifier

General Complications of Humidification

- Bacterial infection in case of stagnant and non-heated humidifier.
- Bronchospasm due to foreign particles and due to dense mist.
- Hypercapnic COPD patients may loose respiratory drive if uncontrolled oxygen is given instead of gas.

General Contraindications of Humidification

- If oxygen delivery device is nasal cannula.

  Because at low flow rates nose provides adequate humidification.
- People with permanent tracheostomy.

  Because adaptation occurs.
- Patients using Venturimask.

  Because water may condense in the entrainment ports and alter FiO_2.

Heat Moist Exchanger (HME)

HMEs are the devices that fit between the airway and the ventilator circuitry. They are commonly referred to as artificial noses. As the exhaled gas pass through the HME, the water condenses on the inner surfaces and heat is retained. The retained heat and moisture are then added to the next inspired breath. Since they conserve heat and water they are called conservers. Since they do not consume electricity to work they are called passive humidifiers. They also reproduce filtration function of the upper airways.

Types

- *Hydrophobic:* Water repellent.
- *Hygroscopic:* Water attractant.

Indications

- During short-term ventilation.
- During transport of intubated patient.

Contraindications

- Patients with thick, copious bloody secretions.
- When exhaled tidal volume less than 70% as in case of bronchopleural fistula, leaking.
- When temperature is less than 32 degree (hypothermic patients).
- When minute ventilation is greater than 10 LpM.
- Cannot be used in dehydrated patients.

Advantages

- Inexpensive, easy to use, small light weight, reliable, simple in design.
- No danger of over hydration, hyperthermia, burns, electric shock.
- Eliminate condensation of water.

Disadvantages

- Limited humidity.
- Temperature preservation not significant.
- Increases dead space in the circuit.

Chapter 20

Nebuliser

DEFINITION

Nebuliser are the instruments which generate aerosol particles of uniform size less than 30 microns in diameter. Aerosol is the suspension of liquid particles in gaseous state.

Types

Bland Aerosol: Delivery of sterile water: It can be hypotonic, isotonic, hypertonic saline.

Therapeutic Aerosol: Delivery of therapeutic dose of selected agents.

Deposition Mechanism

There are different ways by which airborne particles can deposit in the respiratory tract. The five most important ways are **sedimentation, impaction, Brownian diffusion, interception** and **electrostatic precipitation.** In this, interception and electrostatic precipitation does not account for nebulisation mechanisms. The five ways of deposition are summarized in Figures 20.1 and 20.2 and are discussed below.

1. Sedimentation

Sedimentation represents deposition caused by gravity. The chance of particle deposition in the respiratory tract by sedimentation increases as the particle size, particle density, and length of time (residence time) spent in the airway increase. Airway residence time increases as the breathing rate slows. During breath hold in nebulisation always facilitate sedimentation. Respiratory tract deposition by sedimentation is important for particles with an aerodynamic diameter greater than 0.5 μm that reach the medium-sized to small bronchi and bronchioles, where air velocity is relatively low.

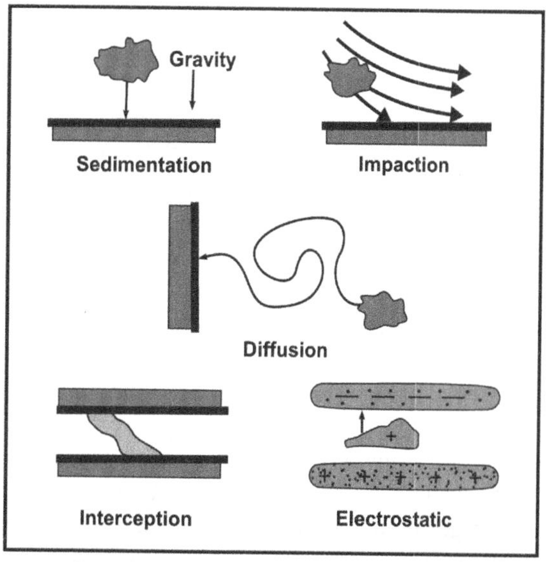

Fig. 20.1: Mechanisms of deposition of particles in the respiratory tract

2. *Impaction*

When the aerodynamic diameter is larger than 1 μm, inhaled particles can deposit in the nose, pharynx and mouth. Deposition by impaction can occur when the particle momentum is too large for it to change directions in an area where there is a rapid change in the direction of the bulk airflow. The chance of impaction increases as the air velocity, particle size, and particle density increase. Air velocity increases as the breathing rate increases. The breathing rate increases as the level of physical activity increases.

3. *Brownian Diffusion*

For particles with an aerodynamic diameter less than 1 μm, Brownian diffusion is a major way for deposition in airways where the bulk flow is very low or absent (e.g., bronchioles and alveoli). With Brownian diffusion, airborne particles acquire a random motion because of their bombardment by surrounding air molecules; this motion can result in particle contact with an airway wall. The displacement sustained by a particle depends on a parameter called the diffusion coefficient, which increases as the particle size decreases. Deposition by Brownian diffusion is especially important for particles with aerodynamic diameters less than 0.2 μm. Particles in this size range may also deposit by diffusion in the upper respiratory tract, trachea, and larger bronchi. Deposition in the respiratory tract by Brownian diffusion is unimportant for relatively large particles.

4. *Interception*

Particle deposition in the respiratory tract can occur when the edge of the particle contacts the airway wall. For elongated particles (e.g., fibers), interception is an important respiratory tract deposition mechanism. The chance of particle interception increases as the airway diameter becomes smaller.

5. *Electrically Charged Particles*

Inhaled particles can be electrically charged. If so, then they can exhibit greater regional deposition over what would be expected based on their size, shape and density.

Figure 20.2 shows that impaction happens only when there is change in direction as in case of high flow rate or increased respiratory rate. Sedimentation achieves with breath hold or with decreased respiratory rate. Diffusion happens with deep diaphragmatic breath. Table 20.1 summarizes the deposition mechanism, particle size, principle used and the technique to achieve this.

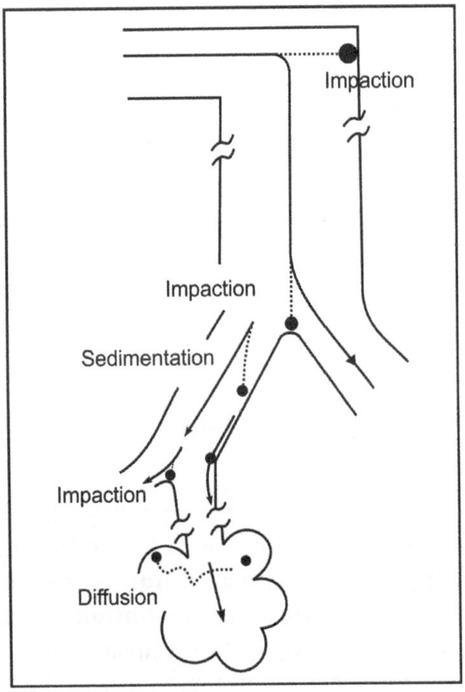

Fig. 20.2: Site of location of impaction, sedimentation and diffusion

Principles

Jet Nebuliser: Uses the principle of Bernoulli's principle.

Table 20.1

Sl No	*Deposition mechanism*	*Particle size*	*Principle used*	*Technique*
1	Impaction	> 1 μm	Momentum	Increase flow rate 15-30 lpm Or increase RR
2	Sedimentation	> 0.5 μm	Gravity	Breath hold or decrease RR
3	Diffusion	< 0.2 μm	Brownian motion	Deep diaphragmatic breathing

As the forward velocity of gases increases, its lateral pressure decreases with corresponding increase in forward pressure. This could also have a baffle incorporated which reduces the size of aerosol particle by removing large particles.

Ultrasonic Nebuliser: Uses the principle of piezoelectric effect. Drugs contained with water in a disc vibrates when ultrasonic waves are passed breaking up the particles held in suspension. In this method heating is not required.

Technique

- Patient is placed in proper body alignment.
- P.D. position can be utilized.
- Patient is asked to take deep inspiration and hold for 2-3 seconds.
- The diaphragmatic breathing can be advocated for maximum effect or maximum distribution and deposition of aerosol in lung bases.
- Proper instruction to the patient should be given (about coughing).

Aerosol Drug Delivery Systems

- Metered dose inhalers.
- MDI accessories:
  - o Flow triggered inhalers – autohalers.
  - o Spacers holding chambers.
- Dry powder inhalers:
  - o Rotahalers.
  - o Spinhalers.
  - o Turbuhalers.
- Small and large jet volume nebulisers.
- Ultrasonic nebuliser.
- Hand bulb atomiser.

Metered Dose Inhaler (MDI)

MDI is a small pressurized canister that contains medication (micronized powder) suspended in a volatile propellant, combined with a dispersing agent to which a mouthpiece is also attached. The high propellant vapour pressure quickly forces the metered dose out through this hole and through the actuator nozzle. When activated, the MDI delivers a single dose of drug. The timing from inhalation to activation of MDI is crucial to the success of delivery to the lungs.

MDI Accessory Devices

MDI accessory devices have been developed to overcome the two primary limitations of these systems: hand-breath coordination problems and high oropharyngeal deposition. Accessory devices include flow-triggered MDIs, spacers and holding chambers.

Flow-Triggered MDIs (Autohaler)

The device is designed to eliminate the need for hand-breath coordination by automatically firing in response to the patient's inspiratory effort. The patients flow will deliver the drug dose.

Spacer

A spacer is a simple valveless extension device that puts distance between the MDI and the patient's mouth. This allows the aerosol plume to expand and the propellants to evaporate prior to reaching the oropharynx. In addition, larger particles leaving the MDI tend to impact on the spacer walls. In combination, this reduces oropharyngeal impaction and increases pulmonary deposition. Holding chambers allow the aerosol plume to develop and thus reduce oropharyngeal deposition. However, a holding chamber also incorporates a valve that prevents the chamber aerosol from being cleared on exhalation.

Dry Powder Inhalers (DPI)

In DPI, drug is placed in the inhaler in its powder form, usually contained in a capsule. When inhaler is activated, the capsule is pierced. The DPI is breath activated; inspiration draws the finely milled drug powder into the lungs. Mechanism to expose the drug powder to an air stream, by three common DPI designs: the Rotohaler, Spinhaler and Turbuhaler. Rotohaler and Spinhaler uses a single dose gelatin drug capsule that must be inserted and punctured prior to inhalation whereas the Rotohaler has no moving parts, the Spinhaler disperses the drug by centrifugal force generated by a small rotor. Turbuhaler store from 60 to 200 separate drug doses in channels or blisters which are opened by rotating a grip or thumb wheel.

Small Volume Jet Nebulisers

The gas stream leaving the jet passes by the opening of a capillary tube immersed in solution. Because the high jet velocity produces low lateral pressure at its outlet, it draws the liquid up the capillary tube and into the gas stream, where it is sheared apart into droplets. This primary heterodisperse spray is then directed against one or more baffles. A baffle is simply a surface upon which large particles impact and fall out of suspension, decreasing the aerosol's diameter.

Large Volume Nebuliser

The jet nebuliser is pneumatically driven, using the venturi principle to create an aerosol. Gases from the flow meter, delivered under high pressure are passed through a jet. The large volume nebuliser is particularly useful when traditional dosing strategies are ineffective in treating severe bronchospasm.

Small Volume Ultrasonic Nebulisers

An ultrasonic nebuliser (USN) uses a piezoelectric crystal to create an aerosol. The crystal transducer converts an electrical signal into high frequency (1.2 to 2.4 MHz) acoustic vibrations. These vibrations are focused in the liquid above the transducer, where they disrupt the surface and create oscillation waves.

Hand Bulb Atomiser

An atomiser used the same basic principles, but does not include baffling. Because only a primary spray is generated, atomisers typically produce aerosols suspensions with large diameter. So the particles mainly deposit in upper airways hence it is used for upper airway obstruction.

Table 20.2 summarises advantages and disadvantages of aerosol delivery devices.

Hazards

1. Dry and retained secretions get swollen and block airways completely. This may be seen in beginning of aerosol therapy better to mobilize secretions before and after aerosol therapy to avoid plugging of mucous.
2. Bronchospasm may be induced by foreign particles present in air stream. On observation look for breathing pattern, administer broncho-dilators.
3. Fluid overload in infants and children can take place.
4. Gross contamination by bacteria itself present in equipment carried in suspension leading to increase in chance of infection–pseudomonas.

Table 20.2: Advantages and disadvantages of delivery devices

Device	*Advantages*	*Disadvantages*
Metered dose inhaler (MDI)	Portable No compressed gas source required No drug preparation required Difficult to contaminate Convenient	Significant patient coordination Difficult to deliver high doses Not all medications available Patient should initiate activation Propellants required High pharyngeal deposition
MDI accessories	No drug preparation required Difficult to contaminate Convenient Easily portable No coordination required	Difficult to deliver high doses Not all medications available Patient should initiate activation Propellents required Large bulky
Dry powder inhaler	Less oral irritation and bad taste Little coordination required Breath activated Breath hold not required Difficult to contaminate Convenient Easily portable No propellants	Patient activation required High flow needed Not many medications available Difficult to deliver high doses Can result in pharyngeal deposition
Small volume nebuliser	No patient coordination required No propellants Able to easily mix drugs Easy to administer high doses Continuous administration Little pharyngeal deposition	Requires compressor gas sources Easily contaminated Treatment time lengthy Drug preparation required Expensive Long treatment times Lacks portability
Ultrasonic nebuliser	Small dead volume Quiet Aerosol accumulates during exhalation	Expensive Prone to electrical or mechanical breakdown Not all medications are available Drug preparation required

5. Excess saline; hypernatremia, localised inflammation.
6. Drug re-concentration during the course of therapy.

Drugs Used in Aerosol Therapy

- **Mucokinetic Agents:** This improve the consistence of secretion and dilute the mucus
  - o E.g.: Normal saline are diluted can be used 50% dilution.
  - o Saline has direct effect on muco proteins making the mucous less viscous.
  - o $Na(HCO_3)$ 2 – 4.7% alkaline can also be used.
- **Bronchodilators:** like salbutamol, epinephrine.
- **Antibiotics:** kanamycin, amikacin can be given.

Advantages

- It has tropical administration, so has rapid therapeutic effects.
- Only a small dose of potent drug is required.
- Avoid extra pulmonary side effects.

Disadvantages

- Patient co-operation is needed.
- It is difficult to monitor prescribed drug dose.
- Only a small proportion of drug is retained in the lung.
- If it gets deposited in or a pharynx. It gets absorbed systematically giving to systemic side effects.
- It can cause tracheobronchial irritation and resultant bronchospasm.

Chapter 21

Medical Gas Therapy

INTRODUCTION

Gas therapy is the most common method of cardiorespiratory care. It includes oxygen therapy, carbon dioxide, nitrous oxide, nitric oxide therapy and helium therapy. Only oxygen therapy will be discussed in detail and other gas therapy will be discussed in short at the later end of this chapter.

OXYGEN THERAPY

Oxygen is delivered as drug to the patient for several purposes. It includes short-term oxygen therapy (STOT) or acute oxygen therapy, long-term oxygen therapy (LTOT), hyperbaric oxygen therapy (HBOT) and Topical oxygen therapy (TOT). STOT is delivered at the hospital and LTOT is given in the home. Topical oxygen therapy is used to facilitate wound healing. Hyperbaric oxygen therapy is the therapeutic use of oxygen at pressures greater than I atmosphere (discussed at the end of the chapter).

Definition

Increasing the concentration of oxygen in the inspired air to correct or prevent hypoxemia is oxygen therapy. O_2 administration aims at increasing PAO_2 and thereby increasing PaO_2 and SPO_2 of arterial blood. If supplemental delivery of oxygen is more than 21%, then only it is called as oxygen therapy.

Rationale

- To treat or prevent hypoxemia thereby preventing tissue hypoxia which may result in tissue injury and even cell death. At the tissue level, mitochondrial activity requires oxygen for aerobic ATP synthesis for cellular activity.
- In case of CO poisoning and cluster headache: In this case affinity of Hb to CO can be reduced. The Half life of CoHb can be reduced from 4 hours to 40 minutes in case of oxygen therapy.
- To resolve pneumothorax who do not require a drainage.

Indications

- Treatment of documented hypoxemia
  - o *Adults, children, infants (> 28 days):* If $PaO_2 < 60$ mm or $SaO_2 < 90\%$.
  - o *Neonates:* If $PaO_2 < 50$ mm Hg, $SaO_2 < 88\%$.
- Situations in which hypoxemia is suspected.
- To decrease the work of breathing.

- To decrease myocardial work.
- Temporary hypoxaemia:
  - o Before and after suction.
  - o First time administration of bronchodilator with side effect.
- Prior to heart surgery.
- During exercise.
- Patients with decreased oxygen carrying capacity:
  - o Anaemia, sickle cell disease.

Assessment of Need

- Use of lab measures to document hypoxemia: Hb, PaO_2, SPO_2.
- Based on clinical problems:
  - o CO poisoning, Cyanide poisoning, Shock, Trauma, Acute MI.
- Clinical manifestations:
  - o Respiratory: Tachypnea, Dyspnea, Cyanosis.
  - o Cardiovascular: Tachycardia, Mild hypertension.
  - o Neurological: Restlessness, Disorientation.
  - o Skin: Cool, clammy.

OXYGEN DELIVERY SYSTEMS

Many devices for administering supplemental oxygen are available. When choosing the appropriate technique for delivering supplemental oxygen, one must consider the device advantages, disadvantages, the FiO_2 limits of the device and its appropriateness for particular patients. Following are different oxygen delivery devices:

1. Low flow systems.
2. Reservoir systems.
3. High flow systems.
4. Enclosures.

Low Flow Systems

These systems do not provide all the gas necessary to meet patients total minute ventilation. They entrain gas enriched with oxygen from the natural reservoir and also they entrain air from room air. The reservoir will be nasopharynx or oropharynyx. So they have variable performance on oxygen concentration.

Types

(a) Nasal cannula.

(b) Nasal catheter.

(c) Transtracheal catheter.

1. Nasal Cannula

Nasal cannula is made up of light weight green or white plastic which consists of tubing and prongs that fit into the nose. Prongs are inserted directly to nose. The maximum flow rate is 6 L/m. FiO_2 can range from .24 to .44 (Figure 21.1).

Best Use: Stable patient needing low FiO_2, Home care patient requiring long-term oxygen therapy.

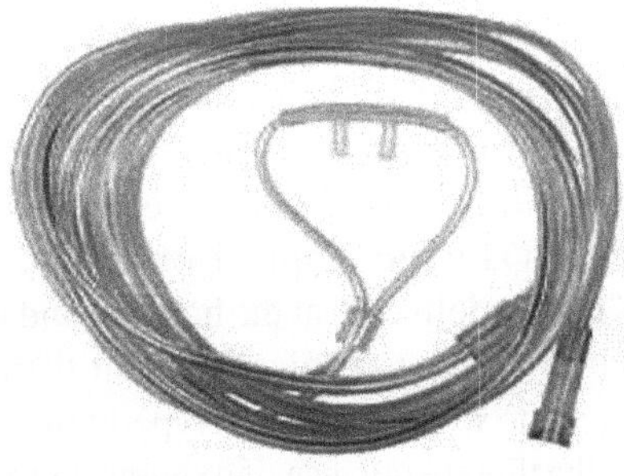

Fig. 21.1: Nasal cannula

2. Nasal Catheter

This catheter has soft plastic tube with several holes at tip and inserted through nose until the tip reaches the oropharynx. It can deliver flow 6 to 8 l/m (Figure 21.2).

Best use: Procedures when cannula difficult to use in case of bronchoscopy.

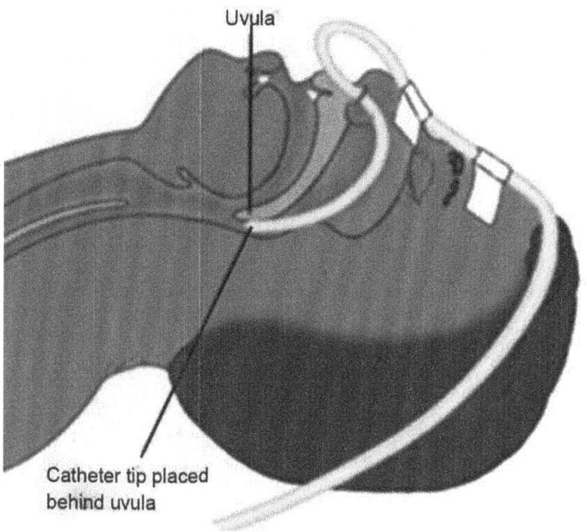

Fig. 21.2: Nasal catheter

3. *Transtracheal Catheter*

This catheter is inserted through tracheostomy opening directly to trachea through 2nd or 3rd rings and flow achieved is 4 l/m (Figure 21.3).

Best Use: Ambulatory patients who need increased mobility or do not accept nasal oxygen.

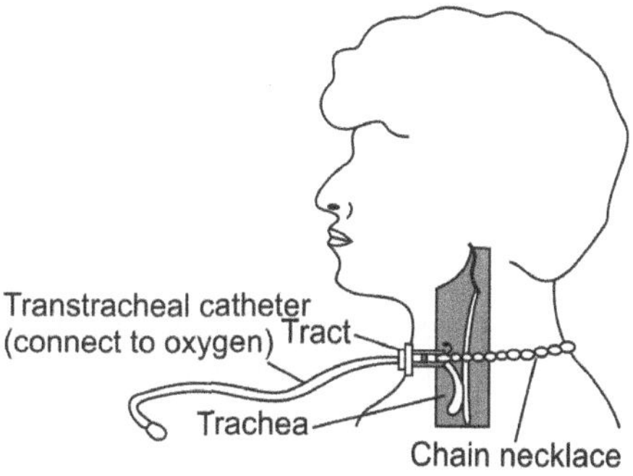

Fig. 21.3: Transtracheal catheter

Reservoir Systems

In this system an artificial reservoir in the form of mask or cannula is added. It can be of two types one with cannula and other with mask.

A. *Cannula*

Reservoir cannula store O_2 between breaths.

Types are nasal reservoir and pendent reservoir (see Figures 21.4 and 21.5).

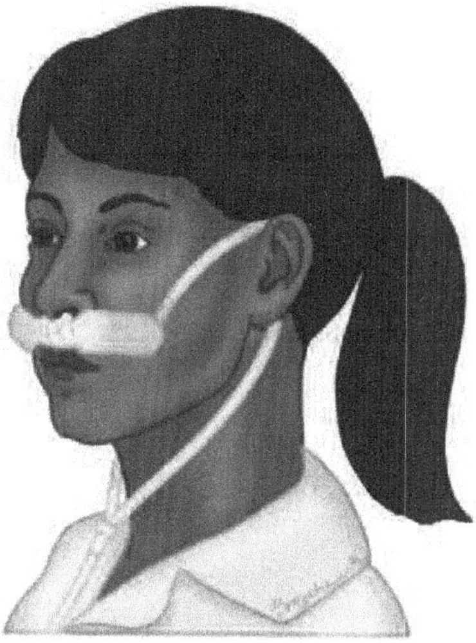
Fig. 21.4: Nasal reservoir

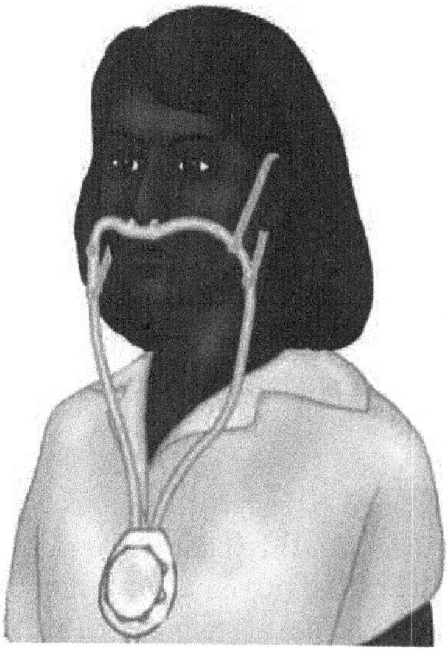
Fig. 21.5: Pendent reservoir

B. *Mask*

It can be of three types:

- Simple mask.
- Partial rebreathing mask.
- Non-rebreathing mask.

1. *Simple Mask*

It covers both nose and mouth. As it increases the size of reservoir, a higher FiO_2 can be delivered. Flow rate varies between 5 to 12 l/m. Through the holes present on the side of the mask, there will be entrainment of room air and release of exhaled gases (Figure 21.6).

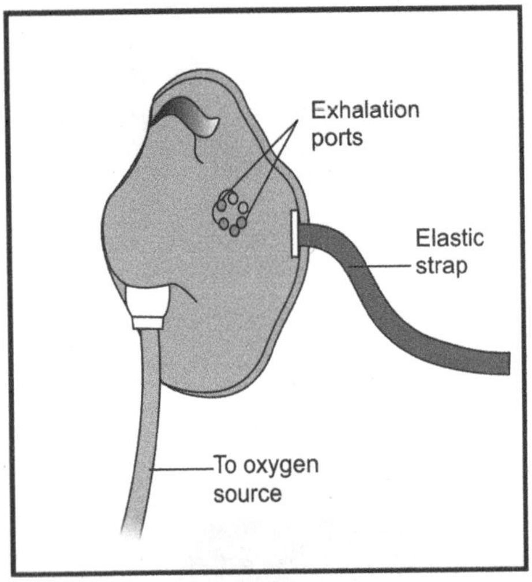

Fig. 21.6: Simple mask

2. *Partial Rebreathing Mask*

The design of this system is similar to simple face mask with the addition of an oxygen reservoir bag. During inspiration the patient draws air from the mask, from the bag and through the holes in the side of the mask. During expiration the first one third of exhaled gases will flow back into the reservoir bag. As this comes from anatomic reservoir, it will be rich in oxygen and contains little CO_2. On the next breath patient will inspire part of previously exhaled gas, along with 100% oxygen from source. It can deliver FiO_2 from .60 to .80. It does not have valves. Flow rate can vary between 6-10 l/m (Figure 21.7).

3. *Non Rebreathing Mask*

The design of non-rebreathing mask is same as that of partial rebreathing mask. But this unit has valves. Valves are present between the reservoir bag and the mask and also on exhalation ports (side port) of the mask. On inspiration, the side port valves close and the valve between the bag and mask connection opens which allow inspiration of fresh air. On expiration, the exhalation port valves open and the valve between bag and mask closes. This prevents entry of air into bag (prevents rebreathing) and also promote release of gas to outside. Theoretically it can deliver FiO_2 of 1 and practically it can deliver upto 0.9. This is because a tight fit of the mask on the face is seldom achieved (Figure 21.8).

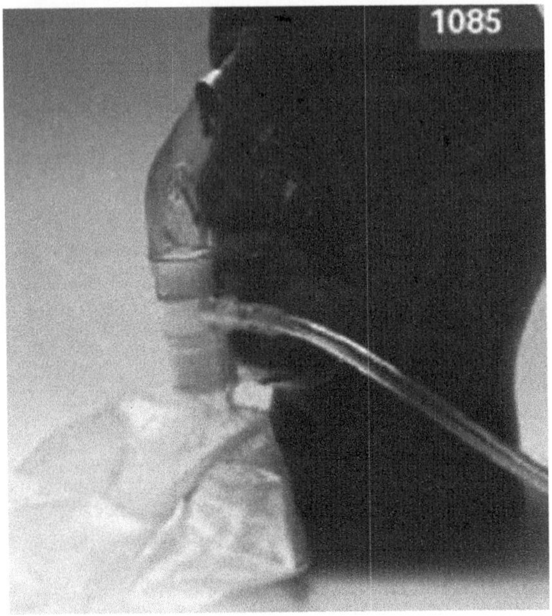

Fig. 21.7: Partial rebreathing mask

High Flow Devices

These systems are those in which the flow of gases is sufficient to meet all of the patients minute ventilation requirements. Compared to low flow system, high flow system FiO_2 fairly remains constant.

Types are:

- Venturi mask.

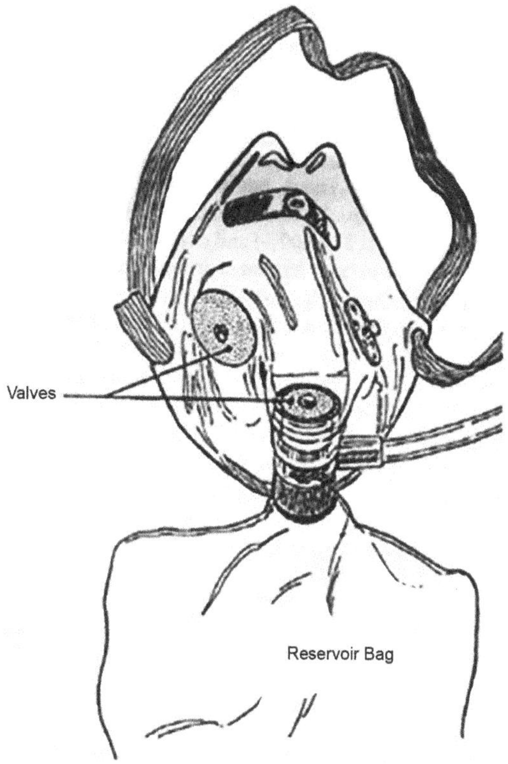

Fig. 21.8: Non-rebreathing mask

- Large volume aerosol system:
  1. High humidity T piece.
  2. High humidity tracheostomy mask.
  3. High humidity face mask.
  4. High humidity face tent.

Venturi Mask or Air Entrainment System

Air entrainment systems direct a high pressure oxygen source through a small nozzle or jet surrounded by air entrainment ports. The amount of air entrained at these ports varies directly with (1) their size and (2) the velocity of oxygen at the jet. The larger the intake ports and the higher the gas velocity at the jet, the more air entrained (Figure 21.9).

Because entrainment devices dilute source oxygen with air, they always provide less than 100% oxygen. The more air they entrain, the higher their total output flow, but the lower the delivered FiO_2. Thus, high flows are possible only when delivering low oxygen concentrations. For these reasons, air entrainment devices function as true high-flow systems only at low FiO_2s. If the flow output from air entrainment device drops below a patient's inspiratory flow, air dilution occurs and the FiO_2 becomes variable.

FiO_2 delivered to the patients is dependent on the size of the nozzle, size of the entrainment ports and O_2 flow. Smallest jet provides highest O_2

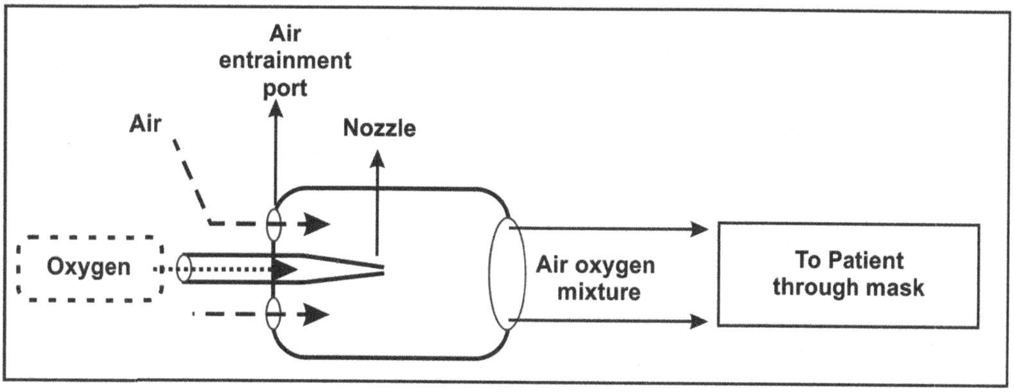

Fig. 21.9: Components of air entrainment system

velocity, thus most air entrainment and the lowest FiO_2 (Figures 21.10 and 11). Table 21.1 lists different types of entrainment port with FiO_2.

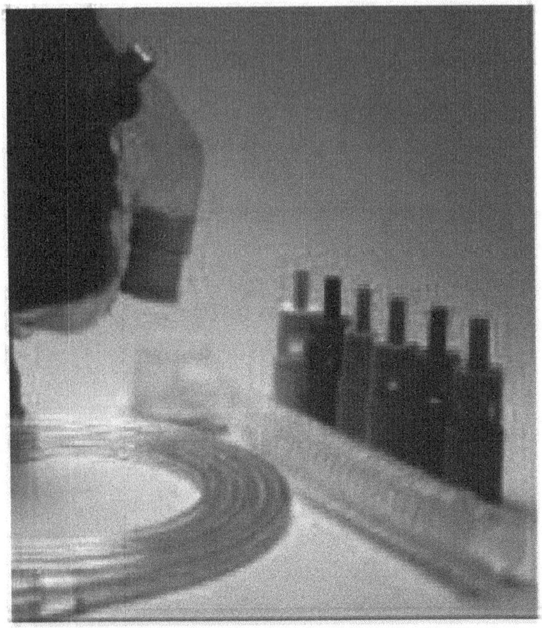

Fig. 21.10: Jet nozzle and entrainment ports (See colour plate no. III)

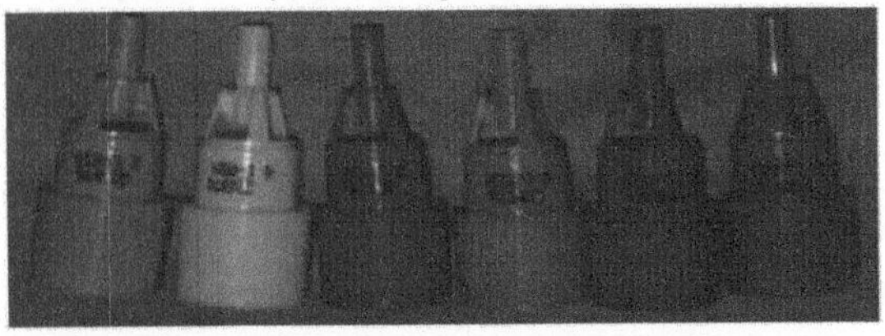

Fig. 21.11: Different entrainment port (See colour plate no. III)

Table 21.1: Colour coding of different entrainment port

Sl No	FiO_2	Colour	Flow L/min
1	24	Blue	2
2	28	White	4
3	31'	Orange	6
4	35	Yellow	8
5	40	Red	10
6	60	Green	15

Large Volume Aerosol Systems

These are the high flow devices, used for administering humidified supplemental oxygen to patients who have an artificial airway which is delivered through T-piece, mask or tent.

High Humidity T-piece

It has three ends in which one end attaches to ET or TT tube, another end attaches to reservoir and third end attaches to oxygen through bubble humidifier. FiO_2 can range from 0.28 to 1.0 (Figure 21.12).

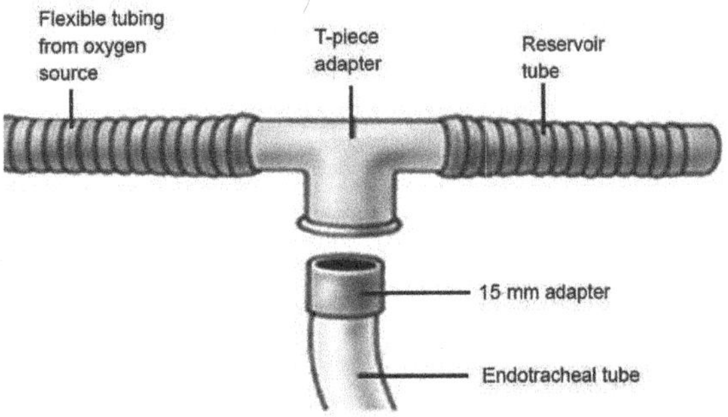

Fig. 21.12: T piece

High Humidity Tracheostomy Mask (Tracheostomy Collar)

A mask is fit over the tracheostomy tube. The hole in the anterior portion of the collar-shaped mask is exhalation port. FiO_2 can range from 0.28 to 1.0 (Figure 21.13).

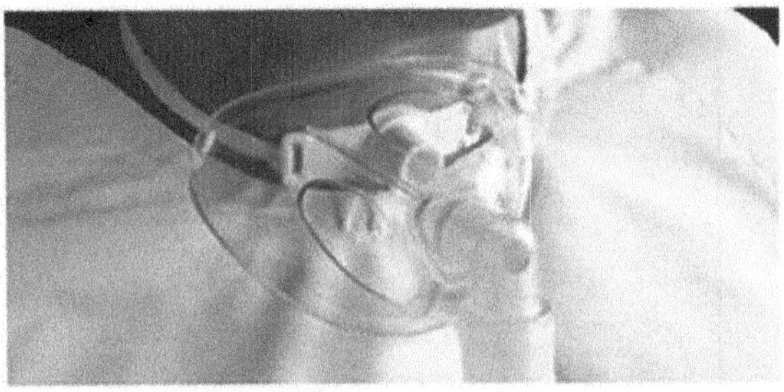

Fig. 21.13: Tracheostomy mask

High Humidity Face Mask

It is similar to face mask with some differences, it is attached to wide bore oxygen tubing and nebuliser and exhalation ports are larger to accommodate larger aerosol particles and high water output (Figure 21.14).

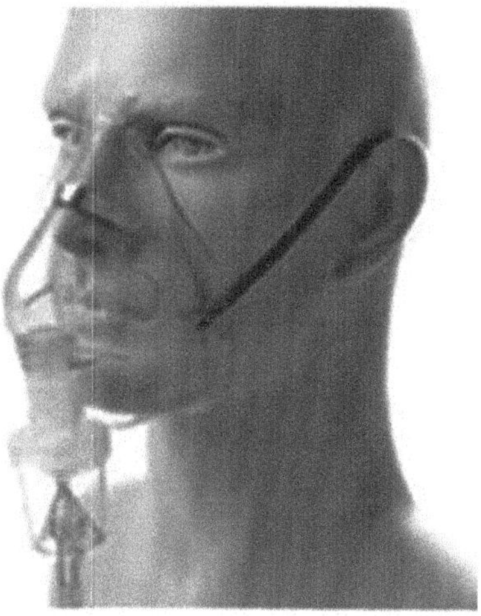

Fig. 21.14: High humidity face mask

High Humidity Face Tent

The face tent is a device that fits under the patients chin, hugging the jaw with top arching over the patients face. FiO_2 can range from 0.28 to 1.0 (Figure 21.15).

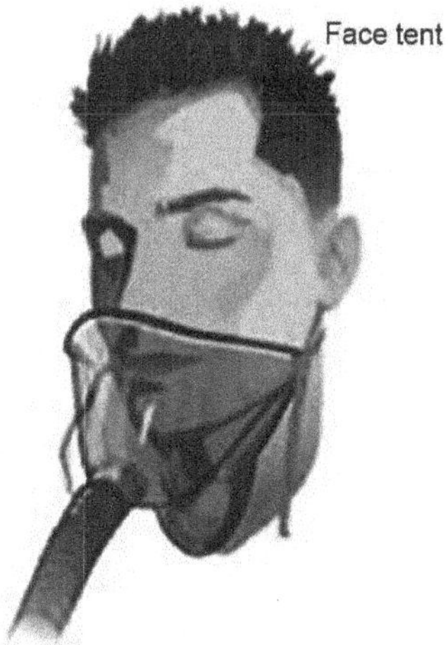

Fig. 21.15: Face tent

Enclosures

Enclosures are generally used only with infants and children. Common types are tents, incubators and hoods.

Oxygen Tents

Tents are air conditioned or cooled by ice to provide a comfortable temperature within a plastic sheet canopy (Figure 21.16).

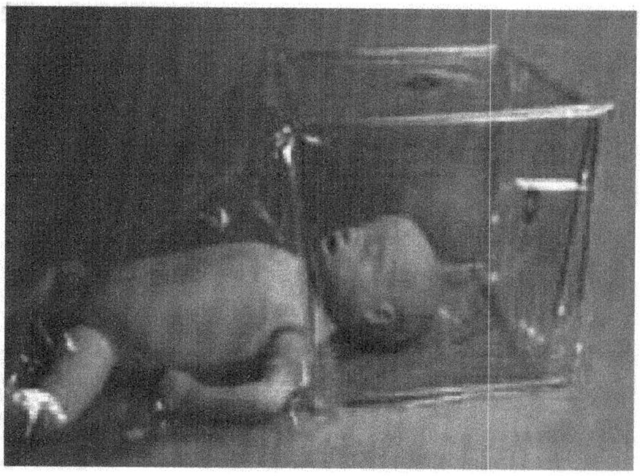

Fig. 21.16: Oxygen tent

Oxygen Hood

An oxygen hood covers only the head, leaving the infant's body free for nursing care. Oxygen is entered to hood by a nebuliser or humidifier.

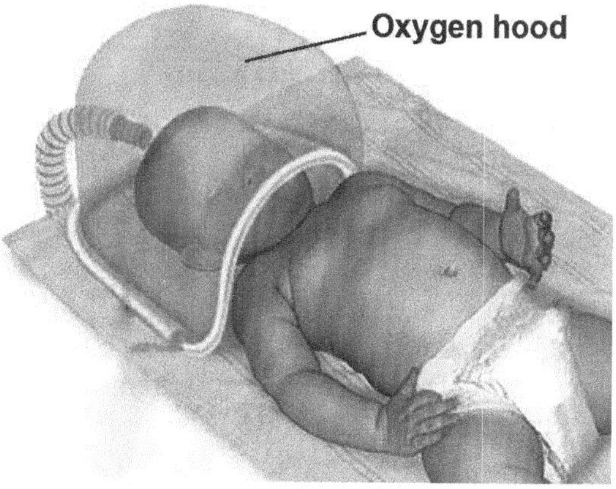

Fig. 21.17: Oxygen hood

Incubators

Incubators are plexiglass enclosures that combine controlled convection heating with supplemental oxygen.

Selection of Oxygen Delivery Devices

- In emergency situation when tissue hypoxia is suspected, patient should be given high FiO_2 through a high flow delivery or closed reservoir system. Clinical examples include cardiac arrest, severe trauma, shock and poisoning.
- In critically ill patients with moderate to severe hypoxemia, patient should be given 60% of oxygen through a reservoir or high flow system.
- More stable patients with mild to moderate hypoxemia, stability of FiO_2 is not critical and can be given through nasal cannula or a simple mask.

Hazards of Supplemental O_2

- Oxygen toxicity.
- Oxygen induced hypoventilation.
- Absorption atelectasis.
- Retinopathy of prematurity.
- Fire hazards.

1. Oxygen Toxicity

Oxygen toxicity primarily affects lungs and CNS. In CNS, it results in Tremors, twitching and convulsions. The exposure of the pulmonary tissues to a high oxygen tension can lead to pathologic parenchymal changes. With the administration of 100% FiO_2 patient complains chest tightness, decreased VC, residual volume, lung compliance. It may also result in bronchopneumonia, interstitial oedema, destruction of type 1 and 2 cells. Tissue injury is due to over production of oxygen derived free radicals that overwhelm the body antioxidants defenses.

2. Oxygen Induced Hypoventilation

Normally carbon dioxide (hypercapnea) is primary stimulant drive for respiration. In patients with chronic hypercapnea CNS response to elevated CO_2 level becomes blunted, then hypoxemia becomes major ventilator stimulus. But administration of high FiO_2 blunts also this drive which results in hypoventilation.

3. Absorption Atelectasis

Normally nitrogen maintains residual volume within the alveoli. During the breathing the high concentration of oxygen, nitrogen may be replaced or washed out of the alveolus. When the entire alveolar oxygen absorbs into pulmonary capillaries, absorption atelectasis occurs. This atelectasis is more likely to occur in the airways that are distal to partial obstruction, because the oxygen is absorbed into the blood at a faster rate than it is replaced.

4. Retinopathy of Prematurity

In neonates and infants, excessive O_2 administration leads to retinal vasoconstriction which leads to necrosis. New vessels form and results in hemorrhage, results in scarring, sometimes retinal detachment and possibly blindness.

LIMITATIONS OF OXYGEN THERAPY

- Directing oxygen into throat does not guarantee its arrival at the mitochondria.
- Oxygen does not improve ventilation directly.
- If hypoxemia is due to a large shunt then oxygen therapy is refractory to hypoxemia especially anatomical shunt.

Oxygen Prescription

Oxygen should be prescribed to achieve a target saturation of 94–98% for most acutely ill patients or 88–92% for those at risk of hypercapnic respiratory failure. The target saturation should be written (or ringed) on the drug chart. Oxygen should be reduced in stable patients with satisfactory oxygen saturation. Oxygen should be crossed off the drug chart once oxygen is discontinued (Table 21.2).

Table 21.2: Advantages and disadvantages of delivery devices

Delivery devices	*Advantages*	*Disadvantages*
Nasal cannula	Patient can eat and drink Well tolerated Low cost Disposable Easy to apply	Unstable Easily dislodged Pressure sore around ear and nose May dry and irritate nasal mucosa Deviated septum may block flow
Simple mask	Light weight Inexpensive Easy to apply Disposable Can use with humidifier Delivery of FiO_2 up to 0.60	Patient may need to remove the mask for speaking, expectoration of secretions Difficulty in placing when Ryles tube in place Drying or irritation of eyes Uncomfortable with facial trauma Block vomitus in unconscious patients
Partial rebreathing mask	Higher delivery of FiO_2 >0.60 Exhaled oxygen from the anatomic dead space is conserved	Insufficient flow rate may lead to rebreathing of CO_2 leads to suffocation hazard Limited access to mouth for eating, drinking, expectorating Eye irritation
Non-rebreathing mask	Higher delivery of FiO_2	Uncomfortable Limited access to mouth for eating, drinking, expectorating Eye irritation
Venturi mask	Delivery of predictable FiO_2 Useful in patients to whom delivery of excessive oxygen could depress the respiratory drive	Limited access to mouth for eating, drinking, expectorating Claustrophobia Irritation to eyes Uncomfortable Noisy
High humidity T-piece	Prevents drying of mucous Helps to thin secretions Accurate FiO_2 can be delivered	Tubing can become heavy with accumulated water Accidentally accumulated water may drain into patients airway during position change
High humidity tracheostomy collar	Prevents drying of mucous Helps to thin secretions Accurate FiO_2 can be delivered	Secretions can accumulate in tracheostomy collar Tubing can become heavy with accumulated water Accidentally accumulated water may drain into patients airway during position change
High humidity face mask	Prevents drying of mucous Helps to thin secretions Accurate FiO_2 can be delivered	Mask is confining Access to mouth for eating, drinking, expectoration is limited Water collected in the tube become noisy Inside of the mask may become wet and becomes uncomfortable
High humidity face tent	Prevents drying of mucous Helps to thin secretions Face tent is more comfortable than simple mask and high humidity face mask for patients with facial trauma or burns	Face tent is difficult to keep in place

Acute Oxygen Therapy

In the acute setting, oxygen should be administered continuously unless hypoxaemia has been demonstrated in specific situations such as sleep, eating or exercise. Acute oxygen therapy is administered in hypercapnic COPD patients, patients with pneumonia or asthma and even in post operative patients. Patients on acute oxygen therapy should have their mask removed for expectoration or other brief reasons. Oximetry is required for prescription, monitoring and withdrawal of oxygen.

Long-Term Oxygen Therapy

Benefits of long-term oxygen therapy in patients are, it can decrease cor pulmonale, increase quality of life, decrease sleep, decrease exacerbations and hospital admissions and improvement of stabilization of disease progression. LTOT should not be prescribed immediately after discharge. Patient should be re-assessed after one month when blood gases are stable. Till that time a temporary cylinder can be supplied for severe hypoxemia. Three systems are available for the LTOT. They are oxygen cylinder, oxygen concentrator and liquid oxygen. Oxygen cylinder contains compressed oxygen delivered through a regulator valve. Oxygen concentrators separate ambient oxygen from nitrogen. Liquid oxygen is stored at absolute zero in thermos containers.

Hyperbaric Oxygen Therapy

Hyperbaric oxygen (HBO) therapy is the therapeutic use of oxygen at pressure greater than 1 atmosphere. Pressures during HBO therapy usually are expressed in multiples of atmospheric pressure absolute (ATA). One ATA equals 760 mm Hg or 101.32 kPa. Most HBO therapy is conducted at pressures between 2 and 3 ATA.

Physiological Effects

1. Bubble Reduction

In conditions such as air embolism and decompression sickness, high pressure exerts a physical effect on air or nitrogen bubbles trapped in the blood or tissues. According to Boyle's Law, high pressure reduces the size of these bubbles and thus minimizes their potential harm.

2. Hyperoxygenation of Blood and Tissue

When a patient is breathing room air, only a small amount of oxygen dissolves in the plasma (about 0.3 ml/dl). At 3 ATA, plasma contains nearly 7 ml/dl dissolved oxygen, a level exceeding average resting tissue uptake.

3. Enhanced Host Immune Function

Oxygen supply to the tissues affects the immune system, wound healing, and vascular tone. A tissue PO_2 of at least 30 mm Hg is necessary for normal cellular function. Lower PO_2 are often seen in damaged and infected tissues. Increasing oxygen supply to these tissues can help restore both white blood cell function and antimicrobial activity especially retarding anaerobic bacterial growth.

4. Vasoconstriction and Reduction of Swelling

HBO causes generalized vasoconstriction and a small drop in cardiac output. Although these changes may decrease blood flow to a region, this is more than offset by the increase in O_2 content. In conditions such as burns, cerebral edema, and crush injuries, vasoconstriction may be helpful, reducing edema and tissue swelling while maintaining tissue oxygenation.

5. Neovascularisation

Although its exact mechanism is unknown, neovascularisation is an essential component of tissue repair, especially in radiation induced injuries.

METHODS OF ADMINISTRATION

HBO is administered via either a multiplace chamber or monoplace chamber. Multiplace chamber is a large tank capable of holding up to a dozen or more people. Because multiplace chamber can achieve pressure of 6ATA or more, they are ideal for decompression sickness and air embolism.The typical monoplace chamber consists of a transparent Plexi-glass cylinder large enough only for a single patient. During therapy, the cylinder oxygen concentration is kept at 100%. Thus, the patient need not wear a mask.

Topical Oxygen Therapy (TOT)

Topical oxygen therapy is a low pressure treatment that applies oxygen directly to the wound site at 1 atmospheric pressure. Compared to HBOT there is less penetration to tissue as there is no additional inspiration of oxygen. It is indicated for diabetic ulcers, venous insufficiency, post-surgical infections, gangrenous lesions, pressure ulcers, skin graft. Treatment lasts for 90-minute session per day for 4 consecutive days, with a rest period of three days. The cycle is repeated until the wound is healed. It is a low cost administration and there is no risk of oxygen toxicity.

Other Medical Gas Therapy

Air

Oxygen and nitrogen can be mixed to produce a gas with oxygen concentration equivalent to air. This medical compressors drive air to the mechanical ventilators to deliver the desired FiO_2. They are also used for powering small volume medication nebuliser.

Carbon Dioxide

Mixture of carbon dioxide and oxygen is used to regulate pulmonary vascular pressures in some congenital heart disorders. Carbon dioxide mixture is also used in membrane oxygenators and to calibrate blood gas analyzers.

Helium (Heliox)

Mixture of helium and 20% oxygen called as Heliox is used to treat large cases of large airway obstruction like asthma. In case of large airway obstruction the flow is turbulent. A turbulent flow makes in less air entry through airways (increases driving pressure thereby reduces airway resistance). So mixture of helium and oxygen lower this driving pressure, more air will conduct through airways. Heliox can relieve stridor, swelling from tumours or burns. It can be used to facilitate weaning by reducing work of breathing. When delivering heliox through a ventilator, the delivered tidal volume may be greater than that set.

Nitrous Oxide (Entonox)

Mixture of nitrous oxide and oxygen is used for anaesthesia purposes.

Nitric Oxide

Mixture of nitric oxide with oxygen dilates blood vessels and it is used for pulmonary hypertension. It improves blood flow to ventilated alveoli thereby reduces intrapulmonary shunting.

Chapter 22

Energy Conservation and Work Simplification

The following problems are commonly experienced by patients with chronic respiratory conditions:

1. Reduced lung functions limiting energy expenditure and functional capacity for meeting daily exertional demands.
2. Dyspnea may induce fear which will further aggravate shortness of breath even when patients attempt the slightest exertion. Patients may become progressively dependent as their activity tolerance deteriorates in time.

For patients with coronary artery disease who have residual cardiac problems following a myocardial infarct, it will be necessary to stress energy conservation. This may be combined with a regular walking program within the limits of their disease.

The use of energy conservation techniques with coordinated breathing and proper body mechanics will help to relieve dyspnea and in turns will enhance patients' ability to cope with daily activities.

ENERGY CONSERVATION

Energy conservation and work simplification refer to completing tasks in the most energy efficient way, in order to have enough energy for the activities you enjoy most. The rationale of the energy conservation techniques is to reduce the unnecessary oxygen expenditure in the body.

STRATEGIES TO CONSERVE ENERGY

Three approaches used here are:

1. Increased awareness on how activity is performed.
2. Modification of activity or use of assistive devices.
3. Compensation by alternative methods or increase dependence on others.

Increased Awareness

It's been observed that COPD patients move rapidly, hold their extremities and trunk in stiff, rigid posture and absence of swinging of arms noted during walking. This pattern results in utilization of more energy compared to relaxed way of walking. Breath holding or shallow breathing during exertion they makes make them more breathless.

So the patient should be instructed to coordinate breathing pattern with movements. Movements that compresses abdominal or thoracic region should be coordinated with expiration. Movements that straighten or enlarge the thorax should be coordinated with inspiration.

Applications of these principles include such things as using pursed lip expiration while bending down to tuck in a sheet while making the bed or bending forward to tie a shoe, and inspiring while returning to the upright position. Other examples would be inspiring while reaching high into a cabinet or/and expiring while the arm returns toward the body.

Activities that have triggered dyspnea in the past should be approached by beginning the diaphragmatic breathing pattern and pursed lip breathing well in advance of the onset of shortness of breath. During stair climbing, standing still while inspiring may allow for a more effective inspiration; climbing is then performed only while exhaling. A brief rest period part way up an incline or stairs may also help prevent the onset of severe dyspnea.

Modification of Activity

Modification of activities of daily living (ADL) involves performing the same activity in a slightly different manner. In this way, energy may be conserved by eliminating unnecessary activities, movement or postures.

All principles discussed in increased awareness of performance should be utilized here as well, such as moving in a slow, relaxed manner, coordinating breathing patterns with activities, and using good body mechanics. Occupational therapists may also be helpful in making patients aware of available assistive devices and assisting with their procurement. Following are the modifications done for the ADLs:

Bathing: The use of shower commodes, shower brushes, and hand-held showers eliminates the need for standing and therefore conserves energy. Bathing aides such as long-handled back brushes and soap on a rope may cut down on unnecessary reaching movements. Drying off after the bath may be made easier by the use of heat lamps or thick, absorbent terrycloth bathrobes to eliminate energy-consuming towel drying.

Grooming: The following suggestions will conserve energy:

(1) Organize the work space to eliminate unnecessary reaching or bending.

(2) Perform grooming activities from a seated position.

(3) Keep grooming routines as simple as possible. Shorter haircuts for women or styles that do not require elaborate hair setting techniques or blow drying will decrease upper extremity work.

Dressing: Many dressing activities may also be performed while seated in a well-organized, central location. Reorganization of cabinet space to eliminate reaching and bending will help conserve energy. Clothes that have front fastenings and are not excessively tight will make dressing easier. Slip-on shoes or shoes with Velcro closures will be easier to manage than laced shoes.

Cooking: The following suggestions will conserve energy: Organize the kitchen to keep frequently used items within easy reach. Perform as many tasks as possible while seated. Avoid lifting and carrying objects. Use a cart to transport items from one area to another, or slide them along the counter.

Cleaning: The following suggestions will conserve energy: Use long-handled cleaning aids to reduce bending and reaching. Organize cleaning equipment to move with you either on a cart or in an apron with large pockets. Avoid lifting. Vacuum rather than sweep. Clean only one room per day. Raise the height of the bed to make bed making easier.

Compensation Approach

When the preceding techniques alone are not sufficient to avoid dyspnea or fatigue during ADL, the transfer of certain tasks to others may become necessary. Tasks may be delegated to other family members or to outside help. Supplemental O_2, if prescribed, may be used during activities that pose difficulty but that the patient still desires to do independently, such as bathing or dressing.

Grooming: Beauty parlours and barber shops may provide hair and nail care on a weekly basis. Often they also employ people who will travel to peoples' homes to provide these services.

Cooking and Cleaning: It may become necessary to hire someone to provide cooking and cleaning services if family members cannot perform these tasks. The use of food delivery services in urban areas or "Meals on Wheels" is also an option.

Shopping: Many grocery stores provide delivery service. In some communities store layouts permit the use of an electric motorized cart, such as the Amigo, with portable O_2 attached, to make independent shopping possible.

WORK SIMPLIFICATION

Work simplification should be simple to learn, but for most people it is not because it requires behavior modification, learning new ideas, changing old habits and adapting work environment.

Energy Conservation and Work Simplification Techniques

1. Establish a Routine

Plan each day to include only what you can really achieve. Gather and arrange supplies or tools for daily activities before start. Leave enough time for each task. Allow 30 min rest period after each meal and after any particular strenuous activity like showering, bathing and exercise and before moving to the next one. Also eliminate unnecessary steps of a task when possible. Plan the daily activity schedule alternating with heavy and light tasks. Always perform minimal repetition of staircase climbing.

2. Pace Yourself

Allow ample time to complete each task. Alter your pace depending on task, temperature and time of the day. Take your time with tasks. Keep a slow and steady pace and not to rush. Listen to your body messages, rest before you are exhausted. Work to music with a slower beat.

3. Sit Whenever Possible

Sit down for your activities whenever possible. Avoid tasks that required prolonged standing, squatting or stooping. Allow placement of your feet flat on the floor and upper extremities should be supported to facilitate the accessory muscles. Avoid tiring and awkward posture that may impair breathing. Try to make habit of relaxed good posture.

4. Eliminate Unnecessary Tasks

Plan ahead and assemble all supplies for a task to minimize extra trips. Straighten bed sheet while still in bed to make bed making easier. Give the tasks to others whenever necessary. Use paper plates and cups when you want to save time and energy. Let dishes air dry. Cut hair short and get a permanent wave.

5. Avoid Strenuous Arm Activities

Avoid straining or vigorous activities using arm motion. Avoid vacuuming, scrubbing, heavy carpentry, washing, heavy gardening, painting walls, digging etc. Avoid raising your arms too high above shoulder level. Let the patient pace himself during other arm activities such as setting hair or strenuous clapping after a performance. Seek consultation from an occupational therapist regarding adaptations to reduce the cost of favourite activities requiring arm work.

6. Keeping Cool

Do activities during cooler part of the day or in the evening. Avoid excessively hot baths. Make slow transitions with temperature such as moving from an air-conditioned building to the hot, humid outdoors, or diving into cool water on a hot day.

7. Watch What You Eat

Avoid stimulants such as caffeine, nicotine, sodium contents.

8. Increase Your Activity Level Gradually

Start easy, with low-level activities at first, taking frequent rest breaks as needed. As you continue to feel better, add a little more each day. Include one or two new activities per day. Gradually increase the duration of your activity periods and shorten your rest periods.

9. Increase Your Activity Gradually

Start easy with low activities at first. Gradually increasing the duration of your activity periods.

10. Avoid Lifting Furniture

Heavy grocery bags, children, the corner of a mattress when making beds, etc. Transport items on a wheeled cart, if possible. Divide groceries and laundry into small, easily handled parcels.

11. Organise Your Work Areas

Keep items that are used most often within easy reach. Store items where they are used most. This does not mean cleaning out all of your drawers and cabinet, it usually means clearing out one or two easily accessible drawers or cabinets and moving a few frequently used items.

12. Avoid Isometric Contractions

Avoid pushing, pulling, lifting heavy items. Avoid breath holding during dressing or other activities requiring concentration. Avoid the Valsalva maneuver.

13. Use Assistive Devices

- Use a shower chair.
- Use long-handled lower extremity bathing and dressing aids.
- Use long-handled tools to avoid bending and reaching (e.g., Reacher, long-handled dust pan, long-handled sponge).

14. Adjust Work Height

The best work height for a table top is about two inches below your bent elbow.

15. Avoid Sustained Position

Change your posture, work height, and placement of objects used in an activity so you are not required to maintain any one position for a prolonged period of time. Otherwise, take frequent short rest periods to ease the stress on your body.

16. Use of Proper Body Mechanics

Instruct the patient to keep his body straight while performing a task, poor posture consumes more energy. Also let them keep their arms straight and close to your body while carrying objects and spread the load between both arms at the same time. Let them support their elbows on table or a firm surface while performing a task to avoid positions that make you tired, e.g., during shaving, peeling potato skin.

Chapter 23

Controlled Mobilisation

Synonym

Progressive Mobilisation.

INTRODUCTION

Before going to the details of controlled mobilisation the words "Mobilisation", "Physical activity" and "Exercise" has to be differentiated.

Mobilisation is the therapeutic and prescriptive application of low workload activity in the management of cardiovascular and pulmonary dysfunction.

Physical activity is defined as bodily movement produced by muscle contraction that increases metabolic demand substantially over the resting state.

Exercise is the form of physical activity that is planned, structured and repetitive.

Mobilisation is given in the acute cardiopulmonary dysfunction, Exercise is prescribed in the sub-acute and chronic dysfunction and Physical activity is the form of behaviour modification program given along with lifestyle modification. Mobilisation is prescribed as both a gravitational stimulus and an exercise stimulus. It optimizes gravitational stress on fluid shifts and central and peripheral hemodynamics. A mobilisation stimulus can cause considerable metabolic demand on acutely ill patients with cardiopulmonary dysfunction. It has also beneficial effects on other systems like musculoskeletal, neurological, gastrointestinal and renal system.

DEFINITION

It is a method of low intensity mobilisation in a slowed and restricted manner.

Rationale

- A simple walking itself increases lung volume and facilitates airway clearance in the patients.
- The upright posture achieved during progressive mobilisation reduces pressure on the diaphragm and encourages basal distribution of air, with natural deep breathing.
- In case of acute illness the patient tends to be recumbent in bed for a great proportion of time. The patient's physical activity is also reduced. The physiological consequences of bed rest is outlined in Table 23.1.

Goals/Aims

- Primarily to exploit the beneficial effects of mobilisation on cardiopulmonary dysfunction.
- Secondarily to explore the beneficial effects of mobilisation on other system such as

Table 23.1: Physiological consequences of bed rest

Cardiovascular system	Decreased left ventricular volume Decreased blood volume Venous stasis Increased resting heart rate Decreased stroke volume Decreased orthostatic tolerance
Respiratory system	Reduced lung volume and capacities, FRC Accumulation of secretions Atelectasis of lower lobes
Muscular system	Decreased muscle mass Decreased muscle strength Decreased endurance
Skeletal system	Bone demineralization
Nervous system	Diminished reflex activity of sympathetic nervous system Slowed electrical activity of brain Depression Sleep disturbances
Renal system	Urine stasis Hypercalciuria Calculus formation
Gastrointestinal system	Constipation Paralytic ileus
Endocrine system	Increased insulin resistance
Integumentary system, skin	Increased sweating, hyperemia Local skin changes

musculoskeletal, neurological, Integumentary, Gastrointestinal and Renal system.

Effects

Following are some of the main effects of mobilisation:

1. Pulmonary System

a. Increased ventilation, perfusion, diffusion, V/Q ratio.

b. Increased mucociliary clearance and quality of cough.

c. Increased volumes and capacities.

d. Increased respiratory mechanics and minute ventilation.

e. Increased flow rate and decreased airway resistance.

f. Increased intercostal drainage.

2. Cardiovascular

a. Increased venous return, myocardial contractility, stroke volume, heart rate.

b. Increased coronary perfusion.

c. Increased circulating blood volume.

d. Decreased peripheral vascular resistance.

e. Increased peripheral blood flow.
f. Increased tissue extraction.

3. *Lymphatic*
 a. Increased lymphatic flow and drainage.
4. *Neurological*
 a. Increased arousal, cerebral electrical activity, postural reflexes and sympathetic stimulation.
5. *Renal*
 a. Decreased stasis and increased urinary output.
 b. Gastrointestinal.
 c. Increased gut motility.
 d. Decreased constipation.
6. *Integumentary*
 a. Increased cutaneous circulation for thermoregulation.

Indications

- **Post-surgical: Post-thoracotomy, Post cardiac surgeries, Post-abdominal:** Here mobilisation may directly jump from lying to sitting, then to standing, then to walking in a fast manner. So, it is called as early mobilisation.
- **Acute neurological conditions:** Stroke, Head injuries, Quadriplegia, Hemiplegia etc.
- **Acute musculoskeletal conditions:** Lower limb fractures, Spinal fractures etc.
- **Acute cardiopulmonary conditions:** Post MI, Pneumonia, Acute exacerbation of COPD and Asthma.

Procedure

Change of positions supine lying to side lying through turning, lying to sitting, sitting to standing, standing to walking with or without assistive devices, then finally to climbing. Also shift of passive exercise to assisted, assisted to free, free to resisted exercise is also included in controlled mobilisation.

Monitoring the Parameters for Progression of Mobilisation

1. *Subjective responses for:*
 a. **Breathlessness:** Borgs RPE scale.
 b. **Fatigue:** VAS scale.
 c. **Exertion:** VAS scale.
 d. **Pain:** VAS scale.
 e. **Discomfort:** VAS scale.
2. *Objective measures such as:*
 a. HR.
 b. SBP and DBP.
 c. RR.
 d. RPP.
 e. SPO_2.
3. *ECG Findings.*
4. *ABG Findings.*

Chapter 24

Exercise Prescription

Indications

Exercise is commonly prescribed for patients with chronic cardiopulmonary dysfunction whereas early mobilisation is given for patients with acute cardiopulmonary dysfunction. Dyspnea and reduced endurance are the primary complaints of patients with chronic cardiopulmonary dysfunction. This may be due to factors limiting exercise tolerance in COPD which is explained below:

1. *Impaired Lung Mechanics*

- Airway resistance is high during expiration, which leads to higher work of breathing.
- Airway tends to close as expiration proceeds; during rest it results in static hyperinflation and during exercise results in dynamic hyperinflation.
- As the lung is hyperinflated diaphragm will be in a mechanical disadvantage which results in early muscle fatigue at low level of exercise.

2. *Inefficient Gas Exchange*

- As COPD patients have hyperinflated lungs but poorly perfused it result in more dead space volume. So patient has to ventilate harder.

3. *Pulmonary Vascular Insufficiency*

- As the right atrial pressure is increased in COPD patients, right afterload is increased. If right heart is unable to respond adequately, oxygen delivery to exercising muscles will be low. This may result in exercise intolerance.

4. *Abnormal Skeletal Muscle Metabolism*

- Deconditioning dyspnea cycle.
- Low level of anabolic hormone associated with COPD patients may result in decreased muscle mass.
- Malnutrition may result in muscle wasting.
- Oral corticosteroid therapy and chronic hypoxemia may lead to maladaptive changes in muscle structure and function which may lead to skeletal muscle myopathy. This may result in peripheral muscle weakness.

Etiology of dyspnea is explained below:

1. Abnormal control of breathing.
2. Inappropriate sense of respiratory load.
3. Excessive ventilation in relation to maximum breathing capacity.

4. Abnormal length tension relationship of respiratory muscles.
5. Abnormal chest wall mechanics.
6. Respiratory muscle fatigue.

Exercise Testing

The parameters of exercise prescription for the patient with chronic cardiopulmonary dysfunction are determined from a clinical exercise test. The purpose of this test is to determine how a patient exercise response differs from the normal and to diagnose the specific limitations to exercise. Exercise testing has to be done for both upper limb and lower limb. In lower limb most commonly a six-minute walk test or shuttle walk test is preferred. But in case of upper limb, a supported upper limb exercise test with bicycle ergometer or unsupported upper limb endurance test to be performed. Whatever the tests administered, HR, BP, RR, Borg RPE scale for breathlessness and fatigue has to be checked prior, immediately and after 3 minutes of exercise testing. Further descriptions of these tests are beyond the scope of this book.

Exercise Prescription

Endurance Training

Aerobic endurance training can be performed at high or low intensity. High intensity training (70 to 85% of maximal work rate) improves aerobic fitness such as VO_2 max, delays anaerobic threshold, decreased heart rate for a given workload, increases oxidative enzyme capacity and more capillarization of the muscle. It also improves exercise endurance. Low intensity training improves the exercise endurance but it does not improve aerobic fitness.

The components of the exercise prescription include types of exercise, its intensity, duration, frequency, course and progression. It can be supervised or unsupervised program.

Lower Limb Training

Mode

For lower limb training walking and cycling is preferred. For combined training daily swimming or canoeing is preferred. Studies have shown that lower limb training improves the exercise capacity, symptoms and quality of life. In the pulmonary rehabilitation outpatient department a rowing machine can be incorporated as it is giving training for upper limb and lower limb concurrently.

Intensity

In case of pulmonary rehabilitation program, training intensity is primarily based on subjective ratings rather than objective ratings used in the cardiac rehabilitation such as karovonens method or MET method or maximal heart rate method. 12 to 15 RPE score is preferred. Even though heart rate is not used for training intensity their age predicted maximal heart rate should not be crossed with exercise.

Duration and Frequency

Initially as the patients have extremely low endurance, duration will be short as 1 to 5 minutes and conducted several times daily. So overall 30 minutes to 40 minutes is achieved daily which has to be conducted 3 to 5 times a week. A warm up and cool down program has to be incorporated along with training program. Warm-up exercise allows for gradual increase in heart rate, blood pressure, ventilation and blood flow to the exercising muscles. Cool down reduces the risk of arrhythmia, orthostatic hypertension and bronchospasm.

Upper Limb Training

Upper limb training is given in both obstructive disorders and restrictive disorders. For upper limb training supported exercise training is given during acute exacerbation of COPD and asthma and unsupported arm training is given during stable phase.

Rationale of Upper Limb Exercise in Restrictive Disorders

When both hands are elevated, the lower floating ribs move outwards. This brings more air entry to the lower lung zones. Also in case of chest mobility exercise where deep breathing is coordinated with trunk and arm movements, the chest wall adhesions are prevented. This increases the expansion of lower lung zones.

Rationale of Upper Limb Exercise in Obstructive Disorders

Upper limb activities commonly require unsupported arm exercise, which poses a unique challenge for patients with COPD, whose upper limb muscles are required to act as accessory muscles of respiration. During supported arm training (distal end of extremity is fixed) these muscle can work as accessory muscles so there is less load on diaphragm muscles and hence less dyspnea. During unsupported arm exercise (distal end is not fixed), the participation of the accessory muscles in ventilation decreases, and there is a shift of respiratory work to the diaphragm. This is associated with thoracoabdominal dyssynchrony, severe dyspnea, and termination of exercise at low workloads, especially in patients with more severe bronchial obstruction. Studies have shown that upper limb exercise training for patients with COPD increases upper limb work capacity, improves strength and endurance, and reduces oxygen consumption at a given workload.

Supported Arm Exercise (Arm Ergometry) or Arm Cranking Exercise

Train at 60% of maximal work capacity. Increase work every 5th session as tolerated. Patient should be monitored for heart rate and dyspnea. Patient should do the exercise for 30 minutes.

Unsupported Arm Training Method with Weight

The starting Dowel (weight) should be 750 g. Lift the dowel to shoulder level for 2 min. The rate of lifting dowel should be equal to breathing rate. Then the patient should rest for 2 minutes. Repeat sequence as tolerated for up to 32 minutes. The patient should be monitored for dyspnea and heart rate. The progression of exercise should be such that weight (250 g) should be increased every 5th session as tolerated.

Unsupported Arm Exercise Without Weight

The most common types of upper limb exercises are mentioned below:

1. Throwing a ball against the wall with arms above horizontal in sitting position.
2. Passing a beanbag over the head in sitting position.
3. Exercises on overhead pulleys in sitting position.
4. Moving a ring across a wire without touching the wire, while arm was above horizontal.

Duration: Each exercise should be performed for 40 seconds followed by 20 seconds rest. Exercises have to be repeated four times in four minutes.

Strength Training

Weightlifting leads to improvements in muscle strength, increased exercise endurance and fewer symptoms during ADL. Lower extremity strengthening may be augmented through aerobic training itself. Upper limb strengthening can be done with low resistance of light weights (dumbbells, pulleys, elastic bands) and progressed first by increasing repetitions (starting with 10 to 20) before adding additional weight. During training physical therapist should monitor breathing pattern and pulse oximetry.

Flexibility Exercise

Patients with progressive chronic respiratory disease loose ROM of shoulder, rib cage. This results in significant changes in posture and reduced mobility. These changes can also be result of inactivity or structural changes of the chest wall, with hyperinflation and adaptive shortening of accessory respiratory muscles. Lower extremity typically loses flexibility because of disuse. Flexibility exercise improves posture, increase ROM, decrease stiffness and prevent injury. Gentle stretching with body movements should be coordinated with breathing exercises. For example, movements that bring full shoulder flexion, back extension and inspiration should be performed with trunk flexibility. Exercise with forward reaching and trunk flexion or with unilateral or bilateral hip flexion should be combined with expiration. Flexibility exercise are also incorporated in warm up and cool down period in the aerobic exercise to relieve muscle tension and anxiety.

Chapter 25

Chest Mobility Exercises

DEFINITION

Chest mobilization exercises can be defined as any exercises that combine active movements of the trunk or extremities with deep breathing.

Goals

- To maintain or improve mobility of the chest wall, trunk, and shoulder girdles when it affects ventilation or postural alignment.
  If a patient with tightness of the trunk muscles on one side of the body will not expand that part of the chest fully during inspiration. Exercises that combine stretching of these muscles with deep breathing will improve ventilation on that side of the chest.
- To reinforce or emphasize the depth of inspiration or controlled expiration.
  A patient can improve expiration by leaning forward at the hips or flexing the spine as he or she breathes out. This pushes the viscera superiorly into the diaphragm and further reinforces expiration.

Indications

These exercises are indicated mainly in pleural disorders, especially after ICD removal for increasing mobility of one side of thorax and preventing adhesions between two layers of pleura.

Types

1. To Mobilize One Side of the Chest

While sitting, having the patient bend away from the tight side to lengthen tight structures and expand that side of the chest during inspiration. Then, have the patient push the fisted hand into the lateral aspect of the chest, as he or she bends toward the tight side and breathes out. Progress by having the patient raise the arm on the tight side of the chest over the head and side bend away from the tight side. This will place an additional stretch on the tight tissues.

2. To Mobilize the Upper Chest and Stretch the Pectoralis Muscles

While the patient is sitting in a chair with hands clasped behind the head, have him or her horizontally abduct the arms (elongating the pectoralis muscles) during a deep inspiration. Then, instruct the patient to bring the elbows together and bend forward during expiration.

3. To Mobilize the Upper Chest and Shoulders

With the patient sitting in a chair, have him or her reach with both arms overhead (180 degrees bilateral shoulder flexion and slight abduction) during inspiration. Then have the patient bend forward at the hips and reach for the floor during expiration.

4. To Increase Expiration During Deep Breathing

Have the patient breathe in while in a hook-lying position (hips and knees are slightly flexed). Then, instruct the patient to pull both knees to the chest (one at a time to protect the low back) during expiration. This pushes the abdominal contents superiorly into the diaphragm to assist with expiration.

5. Wand Exercises

A. Shoulder Flexion and Abduction

Patient should be in standing grasping the wand with both hands a shoulder width apart and lifting the stick overhead. Patient should coordinate shoulders flexion during inspiration and shoulder extension during expiration..

B. Shoulder External and Internal Rotation

In starting position, patient in standing, the patients shoulder are abducted 90 degrees and in internal rotation and the elbow are flexed 90 degrees. Wand is grasped by both hands. During inspiration patient will perform external rotation, the wand is moved towards patients head. During expiration the patient will perform internal rotation; the wand is moved towards waist line.

Chapter 26

Relaxation

STRESS

Stress has been described as the non-specific result of any demand upon the body, be it mental or somatic demand for survival and the accomplishment of our aims. People with chronic lung disease suffer muscle tension from breathlessness, stress and body positions needed to ease their breathing pattern. The stress reaction represents an increase in sympathetic nervous system activity. Stress in a chronic lung disease patient can increase heart rate and respiratory rate. A repeatedly active muscle such as diaphragm needs relaxation in order to return to its resting position after contraction. These patients' accessory muscles have been over used and would have accustomed to muscle tension. The patients would have been forgetting to relax these muscles.

RELAXATION

Relaxation can be considered the antithesis of stress and can interrupt the continuing cycle between physical and emotional symptoms. Complete muscle relaxation is associated with decreased sympathetic nervous system activity, including reduced respiratory rate, O_2 consumption, heart rate, and blood pressure. Relaxation requires conscious control over well-established ways of dealing with tension. Reduction of muscular tension and resting the mind can cause the individual to have a sense of greater control over the body.

Relaxation is facilitated by positioning, sensitive handling and provision of information to reduce anxiety. Deeper relaxation may be achieved by learning a relaxation technique. This can be learned from books, tapes or classes. Relaxation can be achieved by other ways. Participants often have their own ideas, e.g., sewing, jigsaws or for insomniacs watching a lighted aquarium at night. Patient should be warm, comfortable and have adequate fresh air.

Effects of Relaxation

The effects of relaxation on COPD patients are to reduce breathlessness, anxiety, airway obstruction, reduced respiratory rate, reduced oxygen consumption, reduced heart rate and reduced blood pressure.

RELAXATION TECHNIQUES

1. Jacobson Method of Progressive Relaxation (Contrast Method)

Principle

When a muscle is voluntarily contracted the same muscles goes for relaxation. So doing away with residual tension is the essential feature of this method. The physiology of the contrast method is that a strong contraction of a muscle is followed by an equal relaxation of the same muscle or excitation is equal to inhibition.

The technique consists of a sequence of contractions of muscles performed in a **distal to proximal sequence** in each limb or pair of limbs in turn, followed by letting go or relaxation for an equal or longer period of time.

The progressive muscle relaxation technique involves tensing and relaxing specific muscle groups while concentrating on the feelings of tension versus relaxation. Reclining or sitting are postures conductive to relaxing and are therefore recommended during progressive muscle relaxation.

Guidelines

- Select a quiet, dimly lit environment with few distractions for e.g., switch off the mobiles.
- Use bathroom facilities if necessary prior to do relaxation.
- Loosen all restrictive clothing; remove shoes and eyeglasses or contact lenses.
- Take all regularly scheduled medications, including bronchodilators (Depending upon their response, clients may or may not want to use an inhaled bronchodilator. Some find that the bronchodilators ease their breathing, while others experience tremor or tingling sensations).
- Assume a comfortable position so that muscle tension is minimal. Reclining or sitting are postures conducive to relaxing. Your body should be supported in a bed or reclining chair. Small, soft pillows can be used to provide support at the neck and behind the pillows can be used to provide support at the neck and behind the knees. The straining of a muscle group should be avoided. Tense muscles and discomfort interfere with achieving the relaxation response.
- Use whatever methods are effective in controlling coughing. Coughing can be a major impediment to relaxation therapy.
- Use diaphragmatic and pursed-lip breathing (which the client has previously been taught).
- Place a blanket next to the bed or chair in case the client feels cold. (Some individuals feel cold when they relax, while others report unusual feeling of warmth in their hands and feet, from reperfusion).
- Note breathing pattern. Is it fast, slow abdominal breathing. Counting to six, inhale on one and two, exhale on three to six. Take several slow deep breaths, and exhale through pursed lips.

Sequence

The following relaxation technique is based on the principle that maximum relaxation follows maximum contraction.

Feet (One foot at a time): Tighten all the muscles in your foot and toes. Curl toes and point them toward the floor. Hold tense for 5 seconds. Then relax and feel the tension leave your foot. Let your foot become heavy and limp.

Legs (One leg at a time): Tighten all the muscles in your leg and raise the leg up. Hold your leg tense for 5 seconds. Relax and let the leg return to the surface. Let the tension leave your leg so it becomes limp.

Pelvis: Tighten the muscles in your abdomen and buttocks. Hold your muscles tight and concentrate on the tension for 5 seconds. Then let go and relax. Feel the tension leave your muscles.

Chest: Slowly take in a full breath. While holding your breath, tighten all the muscles in your chest and back for 3 seconds. Exhale slowly and completely through pursed lips. Exhale the tension. Feel the muscles loosen up.

Arms (One hand and arm at a time): Hold your arm out straight, tighten your muscles, and make a tight fist. Hold your arm tense for 5 seconds. Relax and let your arm gradually fall to the chair or bed. Feel the muscles from your shoulder to your shoulder to your finger loosen.

Shoulders: Shrug your shoulders and tighten the muscles. Hold the muscles tight, and concentrate on the tension for 3 seconds. Let go and relax.

Neck: Bring your chin down to your chest as tightly as possible. Hold your neck tense for 3 seconds. Let go and relax. Roll your head from side to side in a relaxed manner.

Face: Squeeze your eyes tightly, furrow your brow, and clench your jaw. Hold your muscles tight and concentrate on the tension for 5 seconds. Let go and relax.

2. Mitchell Method of Relaxation

Principle

Stress causes a patient to adapt a posture. So the muscles controlling these posture are tensed to maintain the same. According to Sherrington's law of reciprocal innervation, if one group of muscles is voluntarily contracted the opposite group relaxes. The antagonistic groups of muscles always relax reciprocally and equally to the contraction of the agonist groups of muscles. Tension will be relieved by contraction of the antagonistic muscles. In this technique, the muscles which will take the patient out of the tense posture are those which are required to contract with the consequent reduction in tension in the muscles that are maintaining the tense posture.

Posture of Stress Sitting

- Face frowned, mouth closed and grinding of teeth.
- Raised shoulder girdle, arms adducted and flexed, hands clenched.
- Legs adducted and flexed, crosses on one another.
- Head and body are held flexed.
- Rapid sigh breathing with intermittent gasping.
- Person sits on edge of the chair.

Sequence

The sequence is usually **more proximal to distal** and each part of the body is given three commands as follows:

- To move so that the tense in folded position of the body is opened up.
- To stop moving.
- To let the brain appreciate the new posture making the patient thinks about the new position in which his body component is now resting. Time should be allowed for this and the patient should not be hurried.

Shoulders: Pull your shoulders towards your feet. Stop. Feel your shoulders are farther away from your ears.

Elbows: Elbows out and open. Stop. Feel the open angle at the elbows.

Fingers and thumbs are stretched out with wrist extended. Stop. Feel the finger tips and thumbs feel heavy.

Legs: Roll your thigh outwards. Stop. Feel your turned out legs.

Knees: Move your knees very gently. Stop. Feel your comfortable knees.

Feet: Push your feet away from your face, bending at the ankle. Stop. Feel your dangling feet.

Body: Push your body into support. Stop. Feel your body lying in the support.

Head: Push your head into support. Stop. Feel your head lying on the support.

Breathing: Breathe in gently. Lift your lower rib upwards and outwards towards your arm pits and breathe out easily and feel the ribs falls back.

Face: Keep your mouth closed and drag your jaw down. Stop. Feel your separated teeth. Close the eyes by lowering upper eyelids. Stop. Enjoy the darkness. Smooth the forehead up into the hair. Continue over the top of the head and down backwards. Stop. Feel the hair move.

3. Benson Relaxation Response

Components

Following are the four essential components of this successful relaxation procedure:

1. A quiet environment.
2. A mental device such as a word or phrase, which should be repeated in a specific fashion over and over again.
3. The adoption of a passive attitude (blocking internal thoughts), which is perhaps the most important of the elements.
4. A comfortable position that decreases the muscle tone thereby minimises the work to maintain these position.

Chapter 27

Electrotherapy in Cardiorespiratory Disorders

Biofeedback

Biofeedback refers to the procedure by which the information about the physiological function is feedback into the individuals by means of auditory or visual signals. In asthma biofeedback is used primarily for the ability of subjects to control their airway resistance. Studies have shown that an EMG biofeedback can increase the PEFR by lowering the tension of frontalis muscle as this muscle is a reliable marker for reduced relaxation. The authors explained their findings by the presence of neural reflex composed of a trigeminal nerve afferent pathway and a vagal nerve efferent pathway. The trigeminal afferent would be capable of altering airway resistance through its effects on vagal output. Another reliable measure is total respiratory resistance feedback in asthma was interpreted with an audio output. In this study patients were instructed to lower the tone that corresponded to decreased total respiratory resistance. Studies have shown that patients receiving biofeedback assisted training in COPD demonstrated improvement in exercise tolerance, increased tidal volume, decreased respiratory rate and increased maximal oxygen uptake. In this study, the training includes instruction in pursed lip breathing as well as biofeedback assisted synchronisation of abdominal and thoracic respiratory movements and biofeedback assisted relaxation of accessory muscles and reduction in muscle tension of same muscles.

Shortwave Diathermy and Microwave Diathermy in Pneumothorax

Studies have shown that application of shortwave diathermy or microwave diathermy increases the absorption of air. With the application of diathermy there is increased temperature under the treatment area. As temperature is directly proportional to pressure, there will be increased pressure in the pleural space which increases the absorption. As temperature is increased there will be vasodilation of pleural capillaries which further increases the absorption.

Electrical Stimulation in COPD

Peripheral muscle dysfunction is one of the factor associated with exercise intolerance in COPD patients where they are often limited by limb fatigue. Weakness, atrophy, structural and metabolic changes have been observed in limb muscles, which in turn, can have a negative impact on exercise tolerance. Peripheral muscle dysfunction in people with COPD is characterized by:

(i) reduced percentage of the oxidative fibres (type I) in relation to glycolytic fibres (type IIa and IIb); (ii) decreased activity of most oxidative enzymes while glycolytic enzyme expression is increased; (iii) reduced capillary density or capillary-to-fibre ratio; and (iv) mitochondrial dysfunction. Taken together, these changes contribute to an overall reduction in the oxidative capacity of the muscles of patients with COPD. Patients with COPD are unable to sustain an adequate training intensity and duration because of the rapid onset of fatigue during the initial stages of the exercise. This normally leads to reduced activity or even to the patient being confined to their home or bed, thus accentuating the deterioration of the overall health status of this individual.

Electrical stimulation can be applied to the quadriceps, hamstrings, calf muscles and glutei muscles. Pulse duration ranged from 200 to 400 ms, and stimulation frequency ranged from 8 to 50 Hz. Intensities can be progressively increased from 10 to 30 mA according to the patient's individual tolerance. Studies have shown that electrical stimulation improves muscle function, exercise performance (increased walking distance and increased time to exhaustion in a constant work rate cycling test) and muscle size peak torque. Improvement in muscle function can be due to neural adaptations might play an important role in the early gains in muscle performance observed after ES. ES induced a preferential increase in the cross sectional area of type II fibres and a decrease in the cross-sectional area of type I fibres that did not translate into improvement of muscle mass or muscle function. Hypertrophy of type II fibres might be explained by the preferential recruitment of these motor units during ES. Another potential explanation might be due to a greater potential for hypertrophy since these fibres showed type II specific atrophy at baseline.

TENS to Reduce Breathlessness

Application of transcutaneous electrical nerve stimulation (TENS), a non-invasive modality over specific acupoints (ACU-TENS) has been reported as an alternative mode of management for breathlessness in COPD patients. 45 min of Acu-TENS at bilateral acupoints Ex-B1.These points are known as Ding Chuan in Traditional Chinese Medicine. They are located at 0.5 'cun' lateral to the spinous process of C7 vertebra, were 1 'cun' is the distance between the medial creases of the interphalangeal joints on an individual's middle finger. An improvement in FEV1 and dyspnea score at the end of Acu-TENS treatment was associated with a concurrent increase in b-endorphin level in patients with COPD. TENS settings to get the effect was Frequency: 4 Hz; Pulse Width: 200 micro seconds; Intensity: highest tolerable by the participant. Studies have shown that the effect of single session of bilateral application of TENS for 45 minutes in patients with COPD showed increase in FEV1, 6MWD and decrease in dyspnoea.

TENS to Relieve Pain in Respiratory Conditions

The most commonly encountered situations for the use of TENS in the area of respiratory care are those of rib fractures, Dry Pleurisy and following thoracic surgery where pain inhibits the patient's ability to expand the lung fully and to huff and cough effectively. Conventional or High TENS is used for the relief of acute pain in case of rib fractures or dry pleurisy. This type of application is High frequency low intensity TENS. The mechanism is blocking Aδ by stimulating Aβ fibres. Treatment has to be given for a minimum period of 40 minutes to one hour. By the applications of TENS, patient feels a soothing effect immediately. Following rib fractures or in dry pleurisy electrodes are usually applied above or below the fractures site or over the nerve trunk and along its corresponding dermatome.

Brief or Intense TENS is commonly used for relief of post operative pain in case of thoracotomy. This type of application is high frequency high intensity TENS. The mechanism of pain relief is by peripheral mechanism. Application of intense TENS results in activation of Aδ fibres. There will be peripheral blockage of nociceptor afferent (by blocking the orthodromic transmissions by antidromic conduction of TENS application. Brain perceives pain due to the TENS stimulation not from the painful site. Treatment time administered is usually less than 5 minutes. In case of thoracotomy electrodes are either placed above the site of incision or on either side of incision.

Contraindications include patients with cardiac pacemakers, patients with known heart disease or arrhythmia, and application over the carotid sinus. TENS should not be used over broken skin, or applied over anaesthetized areas.

Chapter 28

Manual Therapy in Cardiorespiratory Conditions

INTRODUCTION

Manual therapy is a method for treating joints and muscle by specific mobilizations, manipulations and stretching. In patients with chronic lung disease there may be lack of movements in cervical and thoracic spine and even in the rib cage itself. A poor biomechanic chest movement and weak respiratory muscles affect respiratory ventilation. To solve inefficient ventilation from thoracic pump dysfunction, thoracic mobility exercise or mobilization techniques can be performed.

Rationale

The movements of inspiration and expiration may be limited by so many factors which may limit ventilation. So manual therapy can correct these factors thereby mobilizing the chest and improves respiratory function. Following are the factors which can limit ventilation:

1. *Decreased Joint Mobility*

Stiff costovertebral joints limit movements of the ribs. The joints are synovial and subject to degenerative changes. These changes often take place early in joints with abnormal mobility, hypermobile or hypomobile. Joints that are not being used through their full range gradually stiffen, with consequent shortening of the surrounding tissues. The joint capsule contracts and causes pain on movement.

2. *Shortened Muscles*

Shortening of the intercostal muscles leads to decreased movement between individual ribs. As the accessory muscles are more used in COPD patients they may go adaptive shortening.

3. *Pain*

Pain is one of the most limiting factors to movement. Pain on joint movement causes the acting muscles to stop working by reflex action. It also causes protective spasm in the muscles controlling the movement. This leads to reduced circulation and more pain or discomfort, and in turn increased tension and shortening of muscle fibres.

4. *Posture*

Faulty posture, with flexion deformity of the spine, will limit the movement of the thorax as a whole and lead to apical breathing. Increased thoracic kyphosis also leads to the neck being drawn forward and to an increased cervical lordosis.

5. *Diaphragm*

Stiffening of the spine leads to flexion deformity, decreased diaphragmatic action and poor ventilation of the lower segments of the lungs with retention of secretions and deterioration of lung tissue.

Indication

Techniques can be administered to both obstructive and restrictive patients. But techniques are more administered in COPD patients rather than restrictive disorders. Following are some of the indications:

1. Scoliosis or kyphosis.
2. Osteoporosis or ankylosing spondylitis.
3. Spinal cord injuries.
4. Skin disease such as scleroderma, multiple sclerosis etc.
5. Myofascial pain or chest pain.
6. Post thoracic surgery for lung or heart operation.
7. Prolonged use of a mechanical ventilator.
8. Chronic lung disease or pneumonia.
9. Prolonged bed rest or ageing.
10. Other factors; pain, posture, diaphragm dysfunction.

Evaluation

General screening of respiratory problems can be assessed from the signs or symptoms of respiratory depression such as tachypnea, use of accessory muscles, abnormal breathing pattern, cyanosis, nasal flaring etc. Following are important points to assess prior to mobilisation.

Observation

AP: Transverse ratio, breathing pattern, kyphosis and kyphoscoliosis.

Palpation

Chest symmetry, flexibility of sternocostal joint and rib torsion.

Examination

Measurement of chest expansion and evaluation of trunk flexibility (flexion, extension, rotation, lateral flexion and lateral flexion with rotation).

CHEST WALL MOBILISATION TECHNIQUES

Either passive or active chest mobilisations help to increase chest wall mobility, flexibility, and thoracic compliance. This relieves both dyspnea symptoms and accessory muscle use. The mechanism of this technique increases the length of the intercostal muscles and therefore helps in performing effective muscle contraction. The techniques of chest mobilisation are composed of rib torsion, lateral stretching, back extension, lateral bending, trunk rotation, etc. This improves the biomechanics of chest movement by enhancing direction of anterior-upward of upper costal and later outward of lower costal movement, including downward of diaphragm directions. Maximal relaxed recoiling of the chest wall helps in achieving effective contraction of each intercostal muscle. Thus, chest mobilisation using breathing, respiratory muscle exercise or function training allows clinical benefit in chronic lung disease, especially COPD with lung hyperinflation or barrel-shaped chest.

In the case of an unconscious patient, as seen in an intensive care unit (ICU) where prolonged treatment is carried out with or without ventilator support, the "Passive Chest Mobilisation Technique" can be performed on the chest wall by a therapist whereas, in the case of a patient in recovery or good condition, the "Active Chest Mobilisation Technique" can be performed.

Towel rolls can be used to mechanically open up the anterior or lateral chest wall. Use of upper extremity patterns will facilitate the opening of individual rib segments. Active or passive stretching can be added after positioning to gain more flexibility.

Anterior Chest Wall Mobilisation

Patient should be in supine lying position. Place a vertical towel roll down the length of the thoracic spine and allowing gravity to pull the shoulders back to the bed. In this position, the anterior chest is opened up, stretching the intercostal and pectoralis muscles for easier facilitation of upper chest expansion. The benefit of this pattern improves ventilation in upper lobes of both lung and also stretches the pectoralis muscle that may tight.

Posterolateral Chest Wall Mobilisation

This technique has many procedures such as trunk torsion, rotation, and lateral bending. It not only affects the ribs and tissue, but also moves the costovertebral and facet joints. This pattern is very useful in order to improve the ventilation around in the lower lobe of both lungs.

Lateral Chest Wall Mobilisation

This technique can be applied in cases of unconsciousness and good consciousness. The technique can be done in side lying, supine and sitting position.

Side Lying Position

Place one or more towel rolls or pillows under the lower chest (ribs 8 to 10) and allowing gravity to open up the upper chest. To determine an appropriate amount of side bending, make sure that the patients shoulder and pelvis in direct contact with the surface, even with towel roll in place.

Supine Lying

Therapist laterally bends the trunk to one side. Arm can be abducted and hand is placed under head to get more flexibility.

Sitting

Patient actively bends to one side. The arm is also abducted in overhead to gain the extra mobility.

This pattern helps to improve the chest wall flexibility around the lower thoracic and improves the ventilation in both lower lungs. This lateral chest wall stretching effects even the thoracic joints either sternocostal or costovertebral joints also.

MANUAL THERAPY TECHNIQUES

Mobilisation of the Ribs

Specific rib mobilisation can be done to free up an individual segments. Technique can be performed in supine lying or prone lying. In supine lying patient places his both hand clasped under the neck, therapist places the hand underneath of patient thorax and pulls the ribs anteriorly. In prone lying, one hand applies counter pressure, while the ulnar side of the mobilizing hand is positioned along the rib, from the rib angle.

Rib Springing

Rib springing is chest compression on expiration, with over pressure downwards and inwards in the bucket handle direction of rib movement then a quick release at end expiration. This may cause a deeper subsequent inspiration, especially when performed slowly and smoothly. It can be done on one rib or more than one rib. It is used in paralysed patients but it is less effective, less comfortable and less safe than neurophysiological facilitation of respiration. It is contraindicated in rib fractures.

Mobilisation of the Facet Joints

The patient is supine with his legs flexed and arms crossed in front of the chest. The operator rotates the patient passively toward himself and fixates the inferior vertebra of the involved segment with his thenar eminence and flexed middle finger over the transverse processes the index finger and thumb is positioned like a pistol grip and it is mobilised. If therapist cannot hold the patient simultaneously while mobilising, a wedge can be used to create space for mobilising spinous processes.

Mobilisation of Costovertebral Joints and PA Glide to Intervertebral Joints

Vertebral joints connect to the ribs and sternum with a complex unit that promotes chest expansion. Although this movement is very hard to observe, it also is very effective for ventilation. Therefore, this joint movement is promoted for improving ventilation (Vibekk, 1991). So the glides are given at these joints.

Mobilisation of Costotransverse Joint

Superior and inferior glide can be given in prone lying. Illustrations are given at the end of the book in appendix section.

Myofascial release techniques to free up restrictive connective tissue on and around the thorax (e.g., scar tissue secondary to areas of surgery or trauma). MFR is also given to accessory muscles like sternocleidomastoid since they will be in shortened position. This technique will inhibit the use of accessory muscles.

Soft tissue release technique in tight muscle groups:

- Neurological impaired patients like Hemiplegia quadriplegia: Often present with tightness in the pectoralis, intercostal and quadrates lumborum.
- Musculoskeletal impaired patients will have more tightness in the neck and back muscle.

Note: Manual therapy techniques should be given by a trained professional in manual therapy. Author acknowledges Prof Pearl-son (MTFI) for sharing his knowledge and photographs on Manual therapy in cardio-respiratory conditions. Illustrations of techniques are given at the end of this book.

Contraindications

- Severe and unstable rib fracture.
- Metastasis bone cancer.
- Tuberculosis spondylitis.
- Severe osteoporosis.
- Herniation.
- Severe pain.
- Unstable vital signs.

Barrel Shaped Chest and Its Cause

Normal anteroposterior diameter to transverse diameter is 5:6 or 5:7. In COPD and asthma the ratio may come down to 5:5. In these conditions there is intrapulmonary air trapping, which depresses the diaphragm downward and inter-costal outward in a shortened position. The shortening of muscle length before inspiration causes insufficient contractile force. Shortness of breath and decreased chest expansion can be observed clinically.

Chapter 29

Patient Education

INTRODUCTION

The three components of physical therapy intervention include communication and documentation, patient/client related instruction and procedural intervention such as airway clearance techniques. The therapist provides direct instructions to variety of individuals including patients, clients, families, care givers and other interested persons. Educational interventions are directed toward ensuring an understanding of the patient's condition, training in specific activities and exercises, instruction in home exercise program, returning to work (ergonomic instruction) and resuming social activities in the community (environmental access).

Definition

Patient education is a planned activity, initiated by a health professional, whose aim is to impart knowledge, attitudes and skills with the specific goal of changing behaviour, increasing compliance with therapy and thereby improving health.

Goals/Objectives

The overall goal of patient education is for the patient to practice health behaviors that promote health, well being, and independence in self care. Other objectives are:

- To enhance patient-clinician rapport.
- To increase knowledge of health disorder/condition.
- To increase adherence to physical therapy treatment plan.
- To decrease health care costs.

Process

Prior to implement the patient education, they should be assessed for type of learning like visual and auditory. Their level of literacy and knowledge on the concerned subject should be assessed/checked. After this queries/doubts/clarifications on the particular topic should be gathered from the patient. Use all these information to design the content for patient education. Next step is to choose the appropriate method of teaching for the patient. For a visual learner the most common methods are videos, demonstration, pamphlets etc. The different methods for auditory learner are lecture or listening to audio tape. Patient should be evaluated for its effectiveness.

Contents

Following are most common contents used for cardiorespiratory rehabilitation:

- Cardiovascular and respiratory anatomy and physiology.
- Cardiovascular and pulmonary disease process.
- Risk factor awareness and modification.
- Smoking cessation.
- Infection control.
- Health promotion and wellness.
- Home exercise program for airway clearance, lung expansion etc.
- Energy conservation and work simplification techniques.
- Cardiopulmonary resuscitation.
- Nutrition and diet such as DASH (dietary approach to stop hypertension) etc.
- Medications.
- Home oxygen delivery systems.
- Sleep management skills.
- Self monitoring of heart rate, respiratory rate and dyspnea.

Chapter 30

Complementary Therapies

Complimentary therapies may help ease breathlessness and stress.

YOGA

Yoga therapy incorporates breathing techniques, meditation, and postures that consume minimal energy and induce physiological effects characteristic of deep relaxation. Studies have shown that it improves lung function and reduced ventilator response to exercise. Yogic breathing promotes breathing awareness, nose breathing and complete breathing sequence of expansion from lower chest to upper chest.

MEDITATION

Meditation clears interfering thoughts from the mind, reducing respiratory rate, HR and BP. Transcendental meditation (TM) is an advanced form of autogenic relaxation, in which concentration on a specific word or phrase, called a mantra, is silently repeated to quiet the body and still the mind. TM is usually performed for 15 to 20 minutes twice a day.

ALEXANDER TECHNIQUE

The Alexander technique is a method that works to change (movement) habits in our everyday activities. It is a simple and practical method for improving ease and freedom of movement, balance, support and coordination. The technique teaches the use of the appropriate amount of effort for a particular activity, giving you more energy for all your activities. It is not a series of treatments or exercises, but rather a reeducation of the mind and body. This technique inhibits muscle tension, which reduces work of breathing and can improve peak expiratory flow and muscle strength.

FELDENKRAIS METHOD

The Feldenkrais Method is a systematic approach to neuromuscular relearning. The method is suited to healthy people who want to increase the flexibility of their bodies and thinking, people with neurological and movement disorders, and those who want to achieve excellence in the arts, sports, or any endeavor. This uses the principle of least effort and is useful for energy conservation.

MASSAGE

It can reduce blood pressure.

IMAGERY

Imagery uses visualization of peaceful scenes, which can achieve a relaxed alpha brain wave state. Finally, guided imagery, or visualization, is a process that evokes mentally many senses to create detailed images, or daydreams, that assist an individual to relax. One of the more common images is walking to a beautiful, happy, and peaceful spot that becomes synonymous with a relaxing and rejuvenating escape, where all of an individual's worries and tensions are let go and the individual feels free.

HYPNOTHERAPY

A means of bypassing the conscious mind and accessing the subconscious, where suppressed memories, repressed emotions, and forgotten events may remain recorded. Hypnosis may facilitate behavioral, emotional, or attitudinal change such as weight loss, or smoking cessation. It is also used to treat phobias, stress, and as an adjunct in the treatment of illness. It reduces the metabolic rate through deeper relaxation. Hypo involves the use of a somewhat altered level of consciousness to achieve a relaxed state. In addition, patients can be given suggestions that help them accomplish specific goals, such as smoking cessation.

AROMATHERAPY

In this technique different oils are smelled which can affect breathing positively and negatively. This significantly alter the breathing pattern.

MECHANICAL REST THERAPY OR RESPIRATORY MUSCLE REST THERAPY

It is the employment of any therapeutic device that performs a portion of all of the mechanical work of the ventilator pump. For chronic fatigued patients, non-invasive ventilation at home may be part of rehabilitation.

AUTOGENIC TRAINING

It is a century-old European method for achieving relaxation based upon passive concentration and body awareness of specific sensations. Its effectiveness has been shown in relieving many stress-related disorders including anxiety, tension, insomnia, and examination stress. Persons with chronic medical conditions ranging from migraine, colitis, irritable bowel syndrome, diabetes, high blood pressure, to thyroid disease and many other conditions have also been shown to benefit from the practice of autogenic training.

Autogenic training employs autosuggestion to achieve the relaxed state. The individual selects the preferred point of concentration for becoming relaxed:

- Rhythm (e.g., breathing in...out...in...out...).
- Sensation (e.g., relaxation, warmth, heaviness).
- Imagery (e.g., imagining a favourite tranquil scene, such as the beach at sunset, and concentrating on being there; or imagining a peaceful descent, as on an escalator, from a place of high activity to one of quiet and rest).

ACUPRESSURE

Acupressure can relieve bronchospasm. Following are the acupressure points:

- CV17: Anterior midline between nipples, level of 4th intercostal space.
- Lu 1: Just below each coracoids process.
- Bl 13: One and half thumb widths lateral to the lower border of each T3 spinous process.

ACUPUNCTURE

Acupuncture points called as Ex-B1 also known as Ding Chuan in Traditional Chinese Medicine. They are located at 0.5 'cun' lateral to the spinous process of C7 vertebra, were 1 'cun' is the distance between the medial creases of the interphalangeal joints on an individual's middle finger. Traditional Chinese medicine presumes that dyspnoea is due to deficiency of flow of 'Qi' (energy). Acupuncture technique may restore the 'Qi' balance and thereby reduce dyspnoea. Takeshige *et al.* speculated that acupuncture points stimulation can modify respiration by influencing the respiratory centres in medulla. Jobst *et al.* and Lau and Jones have hypothesised that acupuncture stimulates hypothalamus which releases endogenous opiates, thereby reducing dyspnoea and improving exercise tolerance. Therefore opiates are prescribed to suppress respiration which modulates the sensation of breathlessness.

Acupuncture may help relieve COPD by reducing bronchial immune-mediated inflammation, and reducing inflammation in general by promoting release of vascular and immunomodulatory factors, improving both airway mucociliary clearance and the airway surface liquid and regulating cytokine production.

Chapter 31

Nutrition for a Cardiorespiratory Patient

INTRODUCTION

Air and food share common pathways during ingestion. They are processed separately and then blend in the blood for distribution and production of energy.

Consequences

- Malnourished people are unable to improve muscle function and exercise tolerance.
- Malnourishment impedes mobility.

Causes

- A normal sized meal can interfere with diaphragmatic mechanics, associated with breathlessness.
- Appetite is reduced with the taste of sputum, smoking, depression and some drugs.
- Exercise limitation and fatigue discourage the patients to prepare healthy food.
- If a patient holds the breath during swallowing meals results in desaturation.
- Salbutamol increases energy demand.
- Oxygen therapy or mouth breathing can dry the mouth.
- Increase work of breathing raises calorie requirement.

Effects of Poor Nutrition

1. Nutritional depletion impairs ciliary motility, aggravates the emphysematous process, erodes muscle, depletes surfactant and increases WOB.
2. Decreased respiratory muscle strength.
3. Decrease exercise capacity.
4. Increases infection.
5. Hinders fluid balance.
6. Can precipitate hypercapnic respiratory failure.

Management

- Clean the teeth and use the mouth wash to remove bad taste in mouth of sputum.
- Meals should be taken in sitting with elbows supported on table to stabilize the accessory muscles.
- Eat multiple small meals.
- Try to include liquid foods than solid food in breakfast.
- Ensure adequate intake of Vitamin C and E to prevent infection, reduce inflammation and mop up oxidants in tobacco smoke.
- Oral feeds should be taken with a glass rather than through a straw to avoid excess WOB.

- Enteral feeds are best given at night to encourage day time eating and nasojejunal tubes improves tolerance.
- Slow continuous infusion prevents excess metabolic activity which can lead to desaturation.
- As supplementary feeds contains concentrated nutrition it can cause bloating and there is also a chance of aspiration.
- Avoid the intake of carbohydrates as it may produce more CO_2 which results in more oxygen consumption and more the patient become breathless.
- Avoid hard and dry foods as chewing these may increases breathlessness.
- Avoid gas forming foods.
- Avoid intake of dairy foods as it may increase the viscosity of sputum.
- Avoid additives, spicy food and caffeine as it may potentiates peptic ulceration.
- Avoid alcohol which increases pulmonary hypertension, hypercapnia in COPD, produces snoring, sleep apnea, impairs ciliary function and immune function.

Appendix

CHANGES IN TRANSPULMONARY PRESSURE GRADIENT

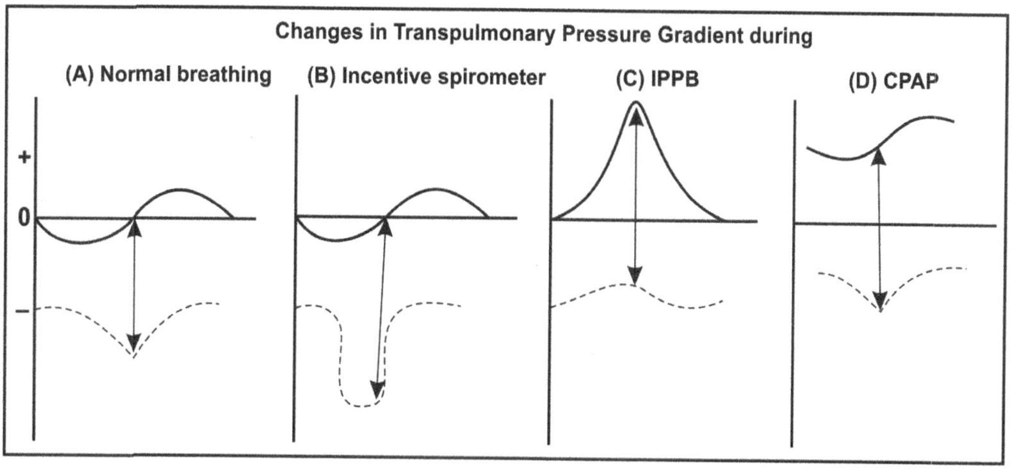

INTERRUPTING THE VICIOUS CYCLE

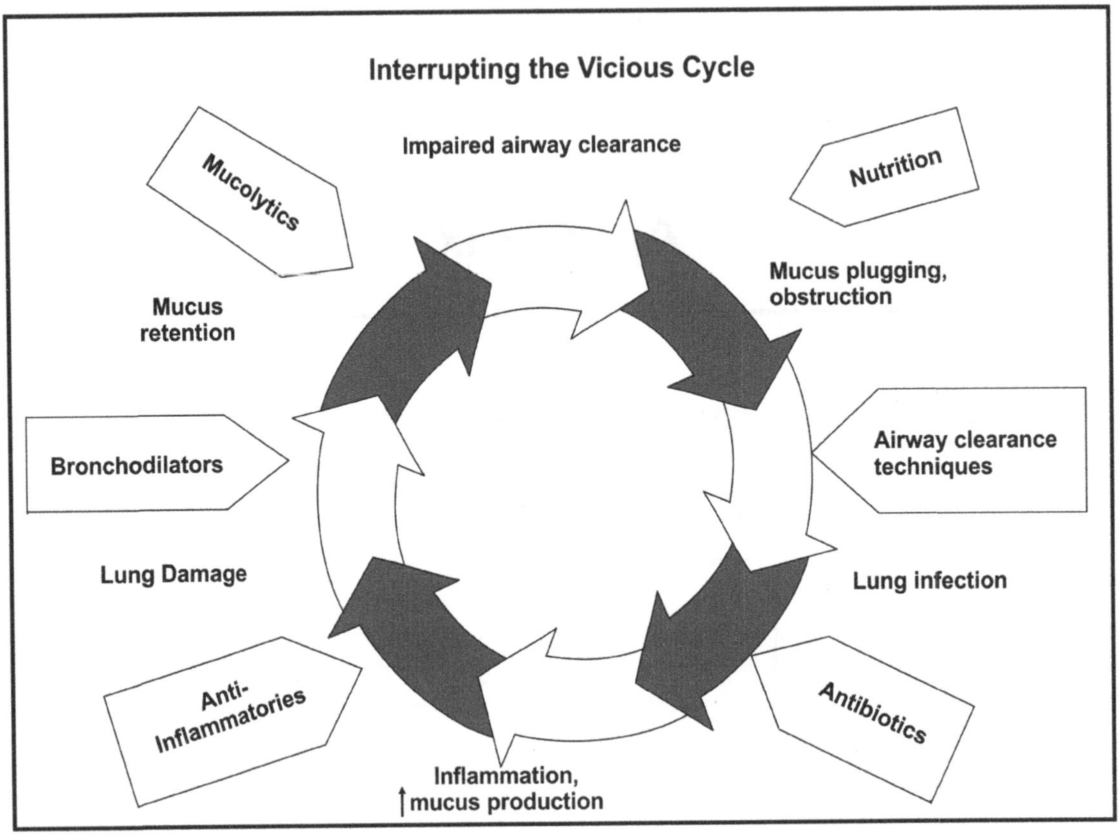

MECHANISM OF MUCOCILIARY ESCALATOR

Mechanism of Mucociliary Escalator

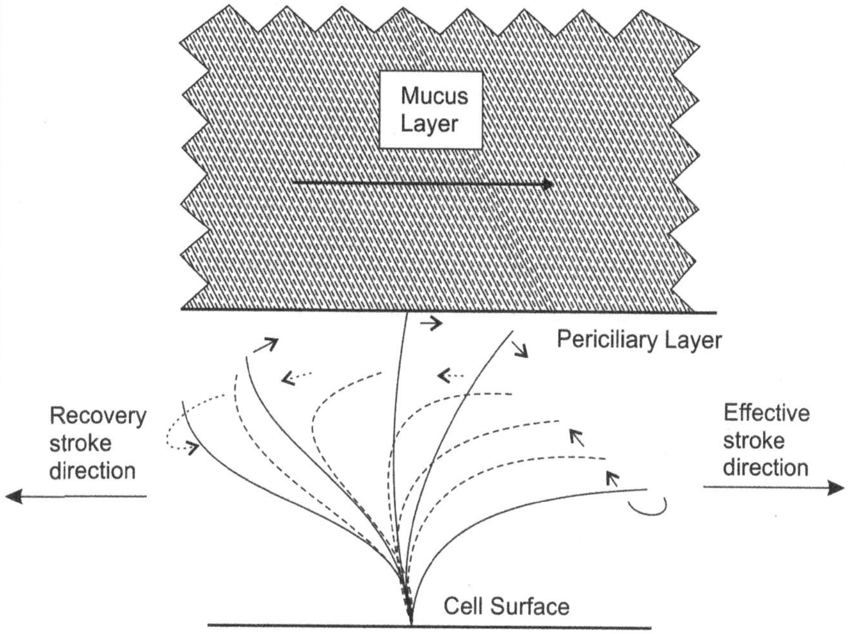

Effective Stroke: (Arrow towards right)
In the above picture it moves the mucous towards right
Recovery Stroke: (Arrow towards left)
The ratio of effective stroke to recovery stroke is 1:3

POSITIONING IN UNILATERAL LUNG PATHOLOGY

(A) Affected side/operated side dependent

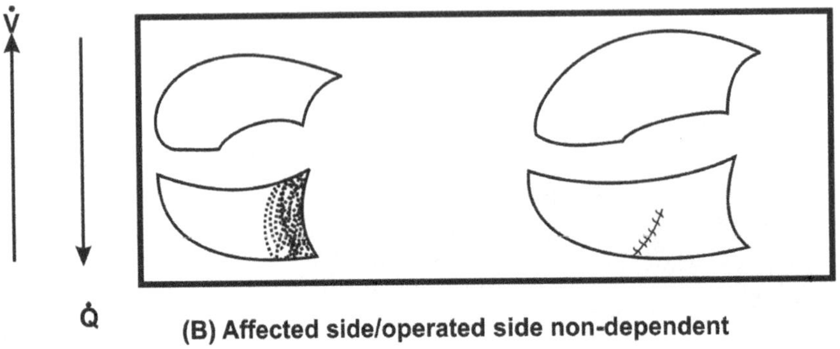

(B) Affected side/operated side non-dependent

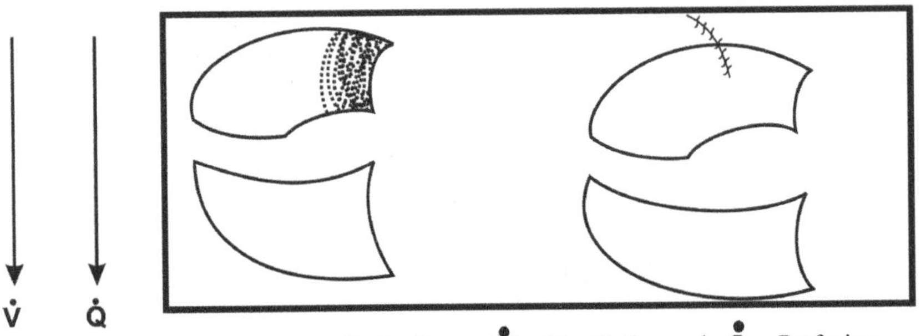

In the figure $\dot{V}$ = Ventilation and $\dot{Q}$ = Perfusion

(as air goes against gravity ventilation will be good in uppermost lung and as blood goes towards gravity perfusion will be good in lower lung)

Unilateral lung pathologies like atelectasis, consolidation, effusions and operated conditions like lobectomy the affected side or the operated side should be uppermost (bad lung up rule). Ventilation and perfusion are usually matched because the better-ventilated dependent lung is also better perfused. For people with one-sided pneumonia, reduced ventilation on the affected side overrides the physiological ventilation gradient. When the patient lies with the affected lung uppermost, the better ventilation of the dependent normal lung is matched with better perfusion. Perfusion is always greater in dependent areas, and V_A/Q match is therefore enhanced in the 'bad lung up' position, sometimes resulting in a dramatic improvement in gas exchange. V_A/Q is usually mismatched if the affected lung is dependent.

As well as optimizing gas exchange, 'bad lung up rule suits other situations. It promotes comfort following thoracotomy or chest drain placement, facilitates postural drainage, and help in improving lung volume when atelectatic lung is positioned uppermost to encourage expansion. With atelectasis, the uppermost areas are stretched and better expanded, even though the dependent lung may be better ventilated because of the compressed alveoli having greater potential to expand and take in fresh gas.

Exceptions to Bad Lung Up Rule

- **Recent pneumonectomy:** When patient lie on operated side, fibrin and fluid deposition takes place in the empty thorax. Hence mediastinal herniation to operated side can be minimized.
- **Large pleural effusion:** Larger effusions are more likely to show improvement of oxygenation with affected side lowermost because this can minimise compression of unaffected lung.
- **Bronchopleural fistula:** In this case any unwanted substances drain into the unaffected dependent lung if positioned uppermost.
- **A large main stem bronchus tumour:** If patient is positioned with operated side uppermost may obstruct the bronchus and cause breathlessness.
- **Whenever patients show discomfort.**
- **Sudden reduction in saturation.**

POSITIONS USED FOR RECOVERY FROM SHORTNESS OF BREATH

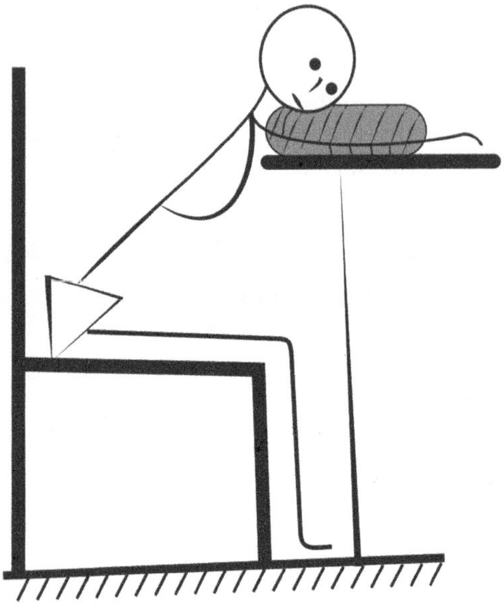

Figure 1: Forward lean sitting (Head and Arm supporting on table)

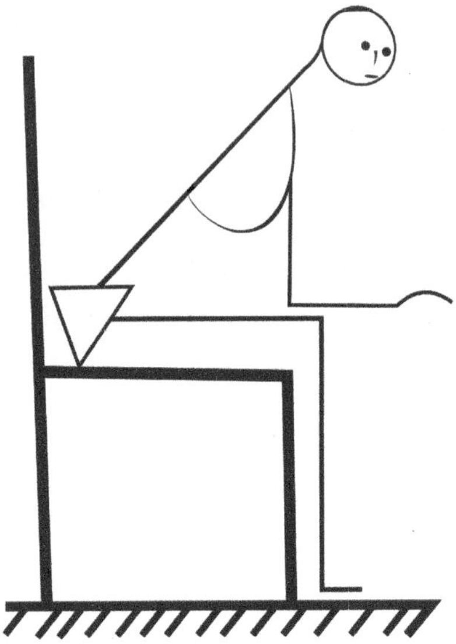

Figure 3: Forward lean sitting (Elbows resting on thighs)

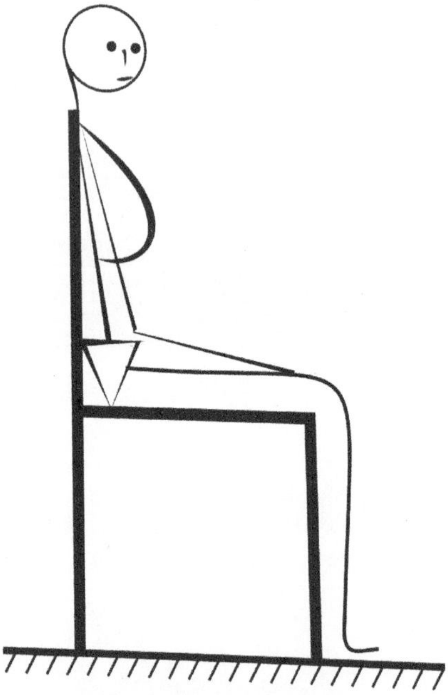

Figure 2: Relaxed sitting

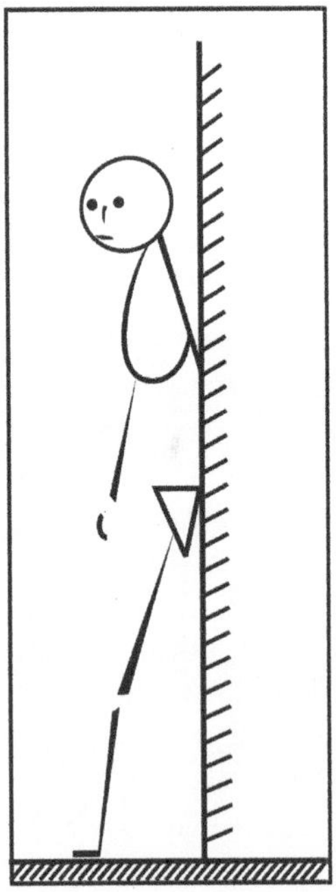

Figure 4: Relaxed standing

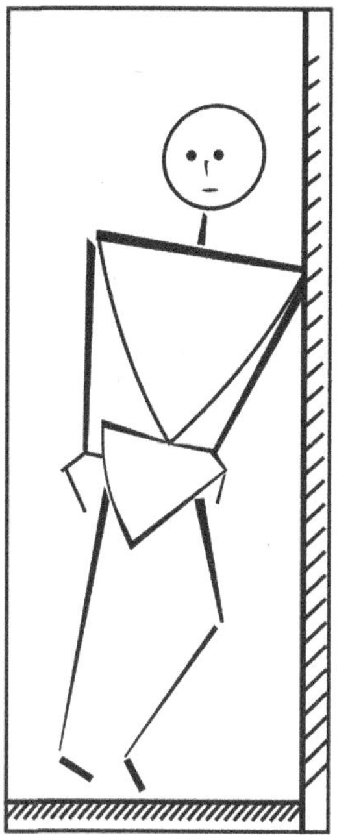

Figure 5: Stride standing (Arms in pocket)

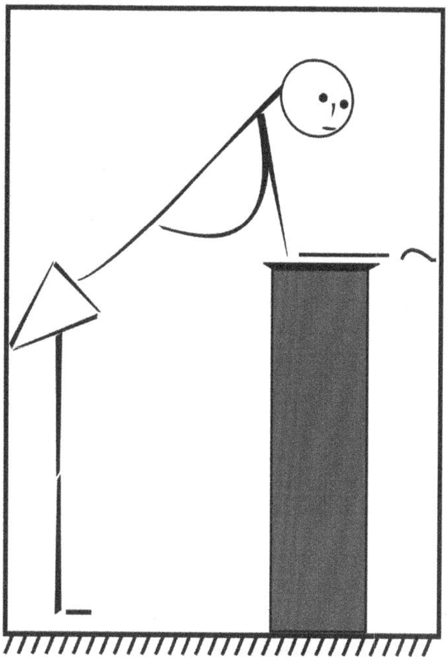

Figure 6: Forward lean standing

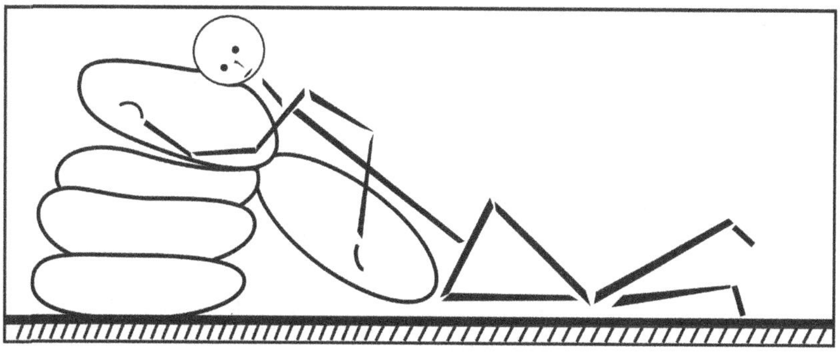

Figure 7: High side lying

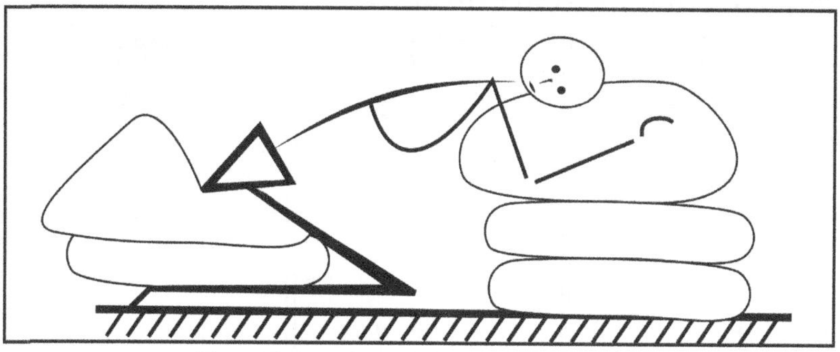

Figure 8: Breathless relieving position for kids

NEUROPHYSIOLOGICAL FACILITATION OF RESPIRATION TECHNIQUES

A. Perioral pressure

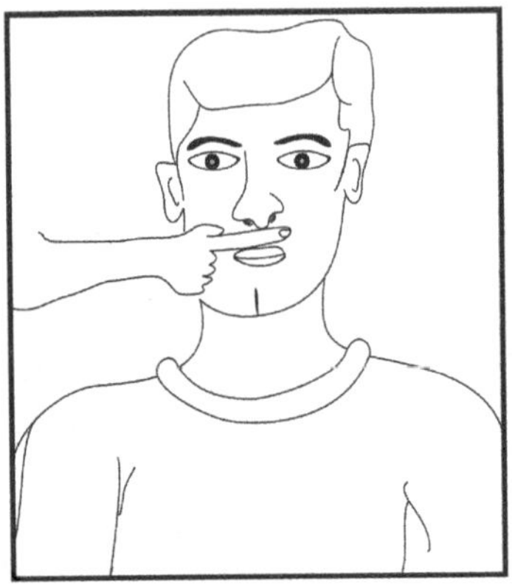

B. Intercostal stretch

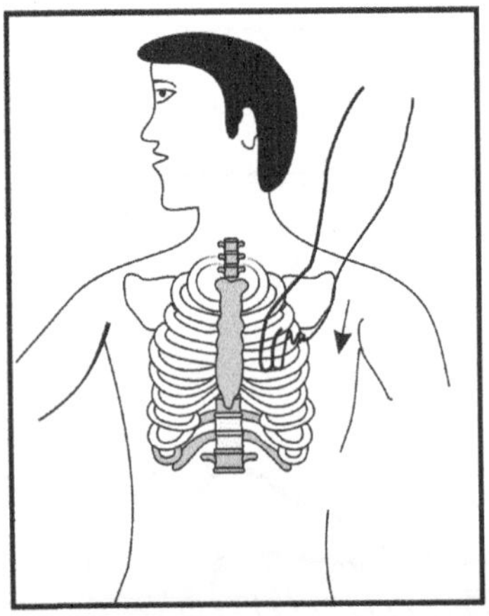

C. Manual vertebral pressure

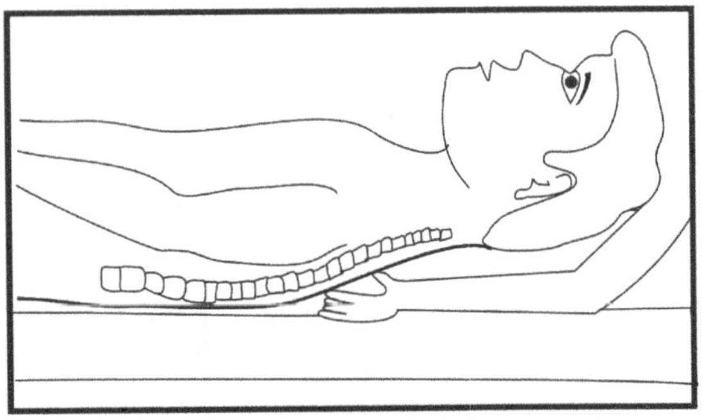

D. Co-contraction of abdomen

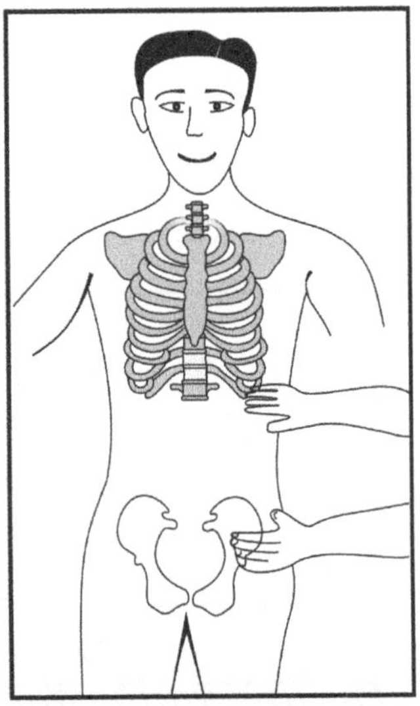

E. Maintained moderate manual pressure

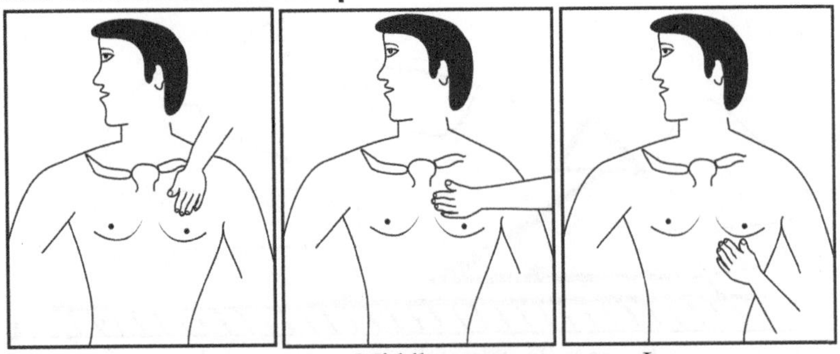

Upper zone   Middle zone   Lower zone

F. Anterior stretch basal lift

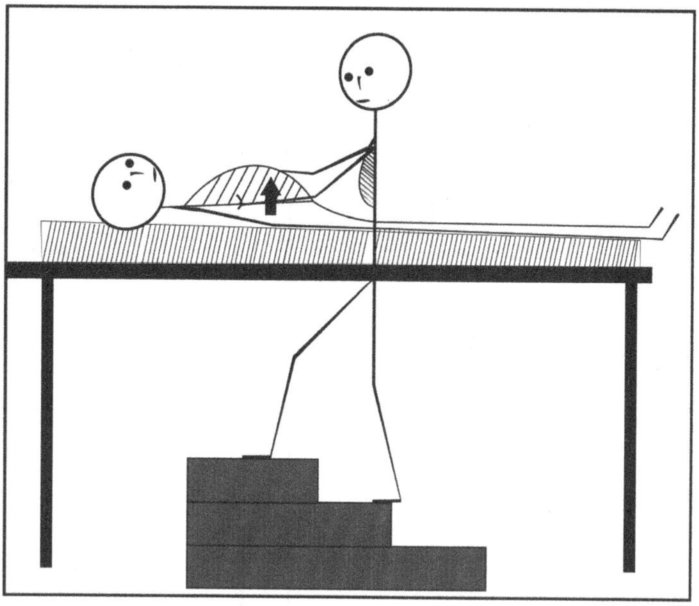

SUGGESTED POSITION TO TEACH DIAPHRAGMATIC BREATHING EXERCISES

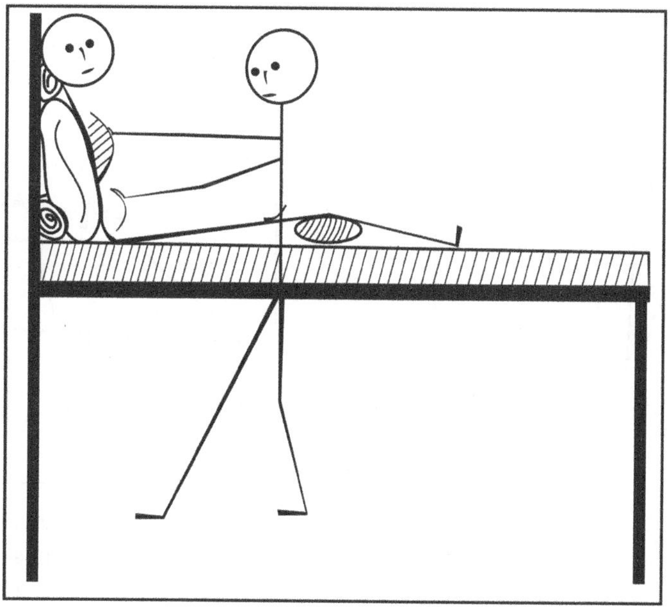

SEGMENTAL BREATHING EXERCISES

Apical costal breathing exercise

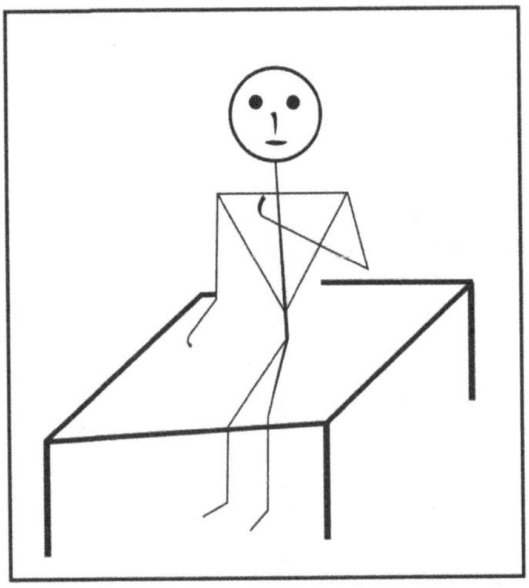

Note: Only unilateral apical costal breathing is done.

Any attempt to do bilateral apical costal breathing results in shoulder girdle elevation and more use of accessory muscle.

Lateral costal breathing exercise (Unilateral)

Hand placement from opposite side

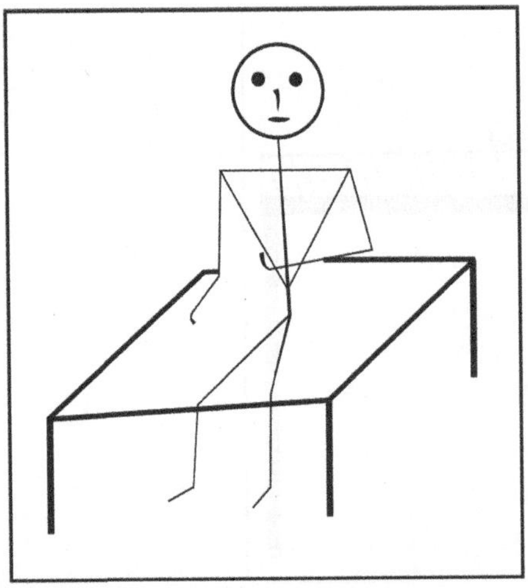

Lateral costal breathing exercise (Unilateral)

Hand placement from same side

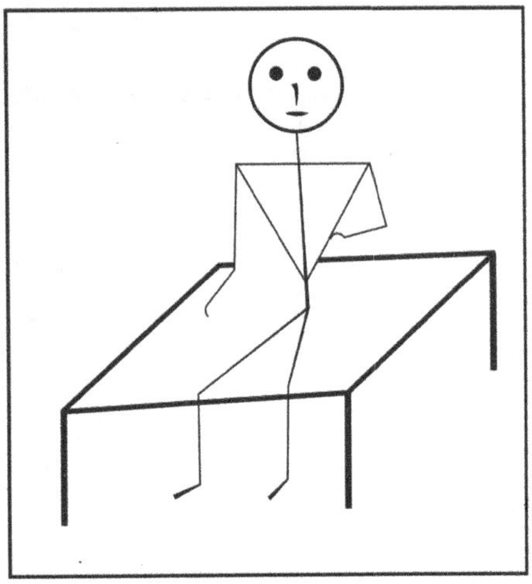

Lateral costal breathing exercise (Bilateral)

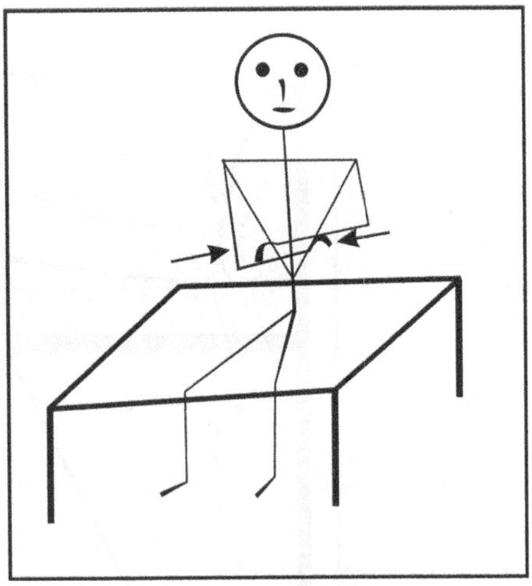

Note: Patient cannot themselves do posterior basal expansion exercises: Therapist has to place hand posteriorly and patient will perform the technique.

POSTURAL DRAINAGE POSITIONS

Upper lobe (both side)

Apico-Anterior

Position: Semi fowlers

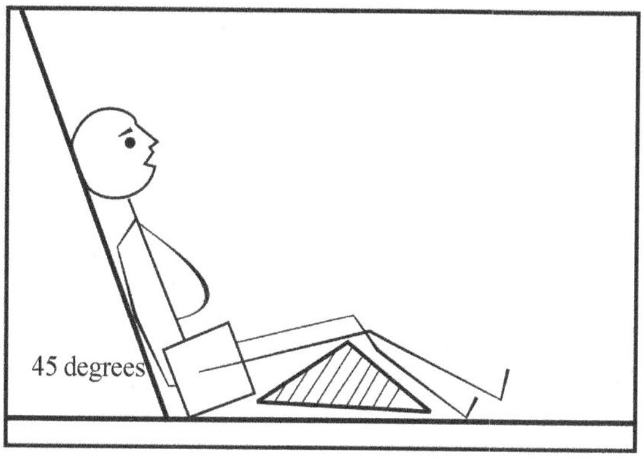

Upper lobe (both side)

Apico-Posterior

Position: Forward lean sitting

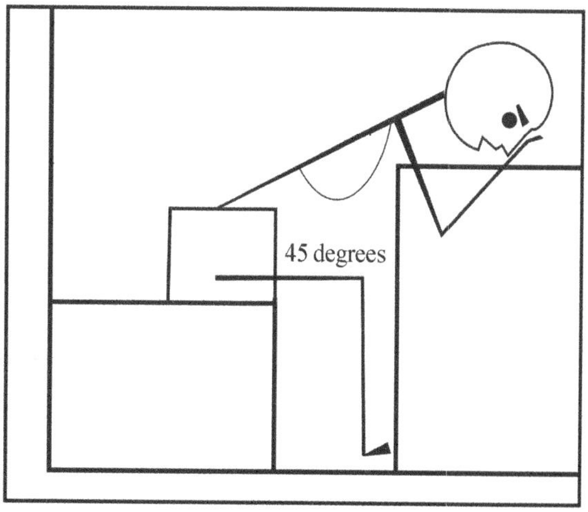

Upper lobe anterior segments

Position: Supine

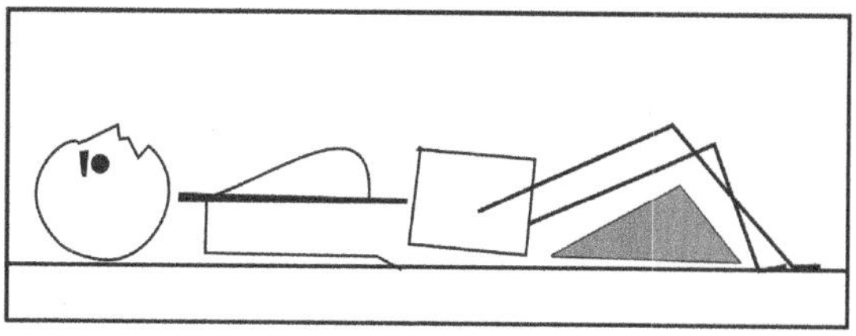

Left upper lobe posterior segments

Position: ¼ turn from prone lying with right arm underneath head and left arm forward with head end elevated 45 degrees

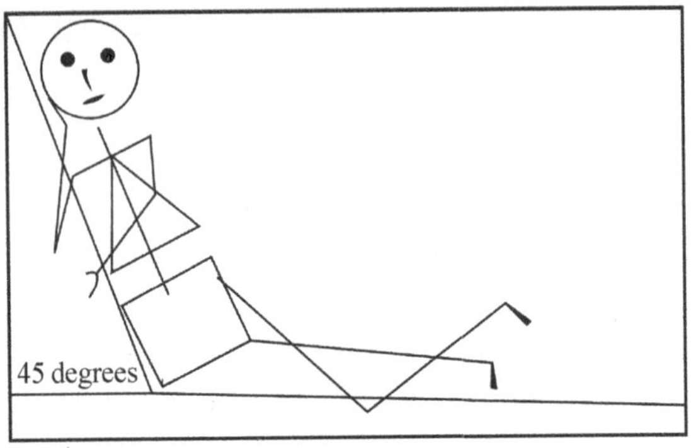

Right upper lobe

Posterior segment

¼ turn from prone lying left arm underneath head with right arm forward without head end elevation

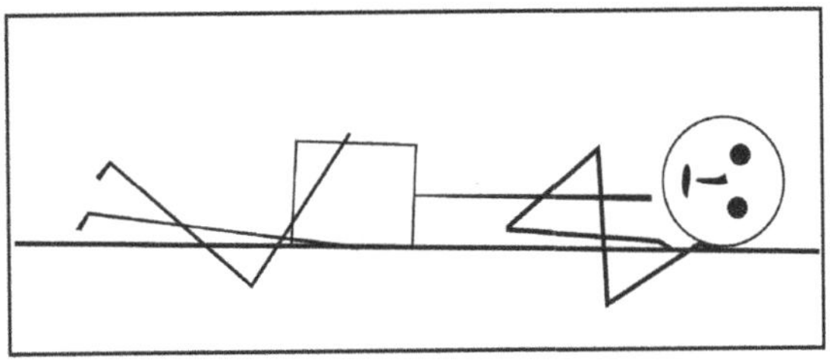

Left lung

Lingula

¼ turn from supine, left side uppermost

14 inches elevation leg side

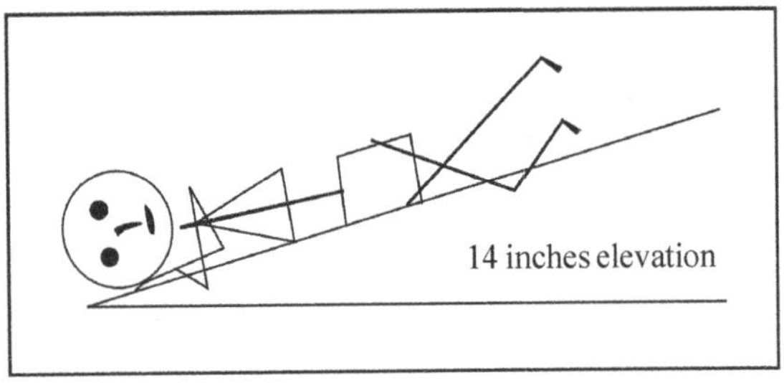

Right lung

Middle lobe

¼ turn from supine, right side uppermost

14 inches elevation leg side

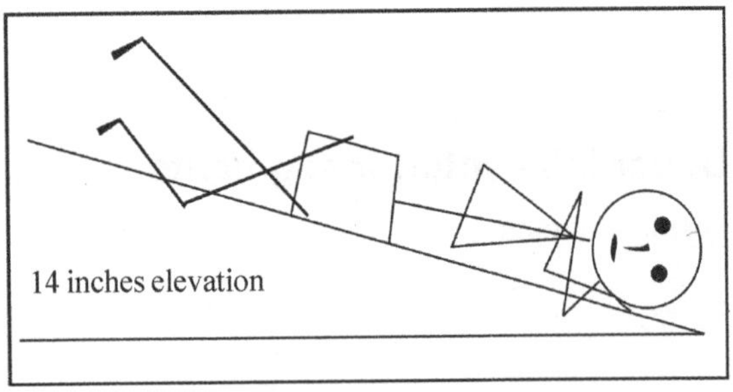

Lower lobes

Apico-basal both sides

Prone lying with pillow under abdomen

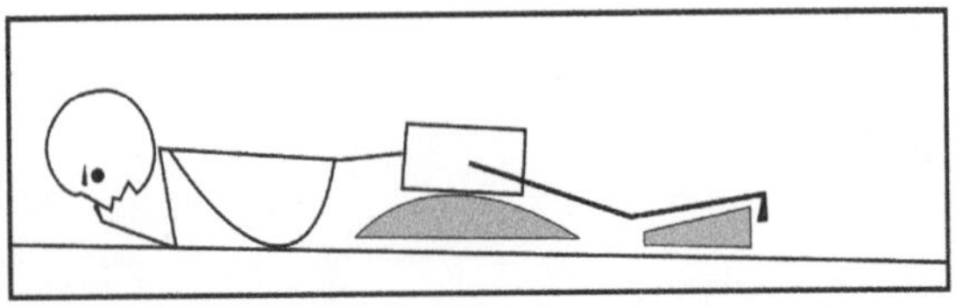

Lower lobes

Anterior basal both sides

Patient supine lying with 18 inches elevation leg end

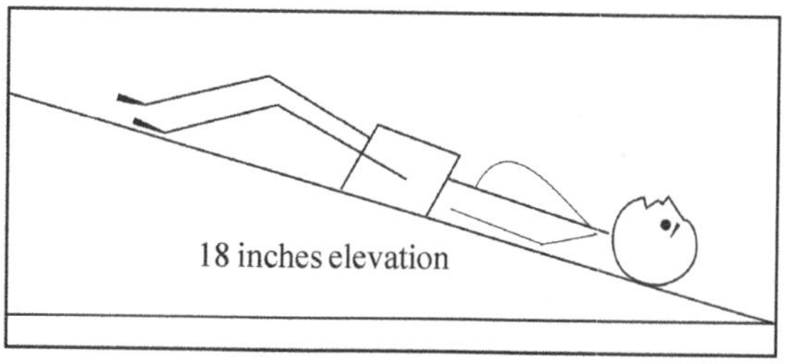

Lower lobes

Posterior basal both side

Patient prone lying with 18 inches elevation leg end

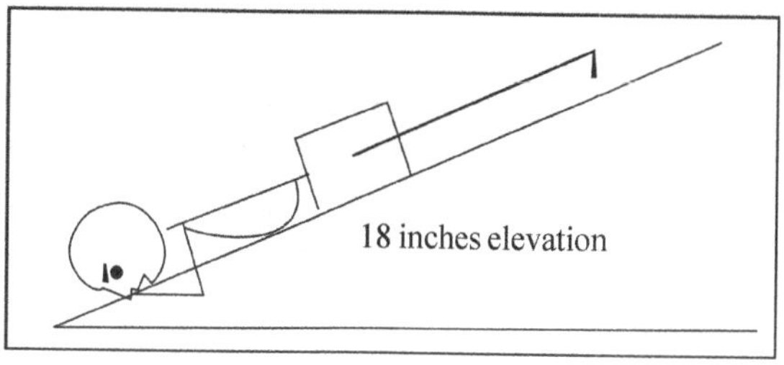

Right lower lobe

Right lateral basal segment

Lying on left side with 18 inches elevation leg end

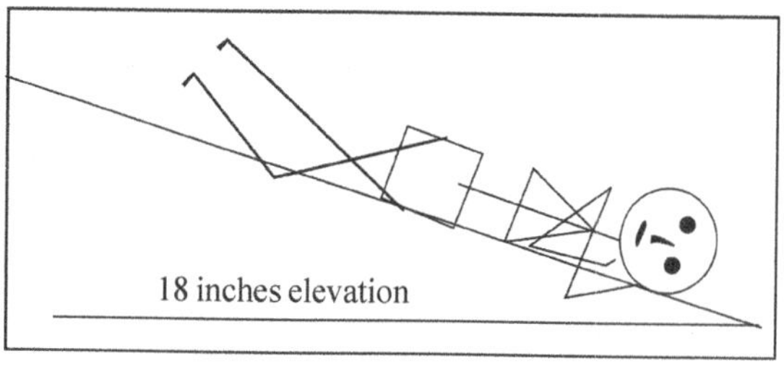

Right lower lobe

Lateral basal of left side and medial basal of right side is drained together

Lying on right side with 18 inches elevation on leg end

Note: Percussions cannot be given for medial basal segments

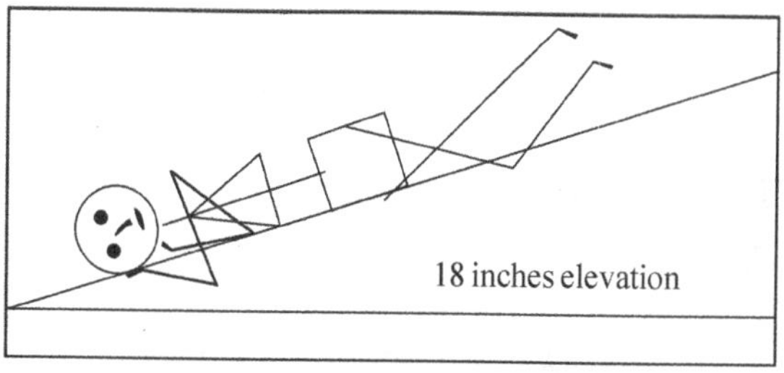

MODIFICATIONS FOR MANUAL PERCUSSIONS FOR NEONATES

Four fingers cupped

Palmar View

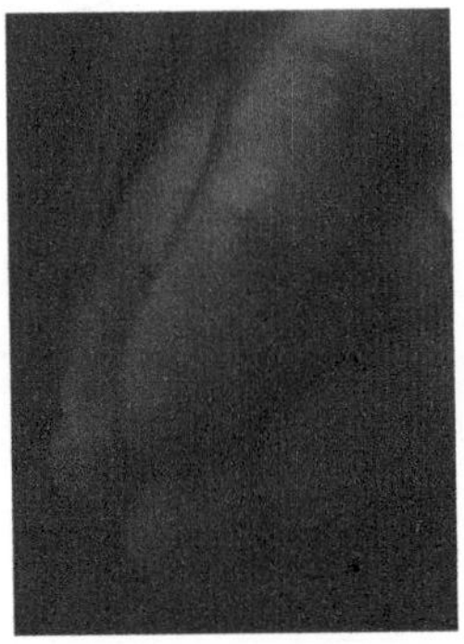

(See colour plate no. III)

Dorsal View

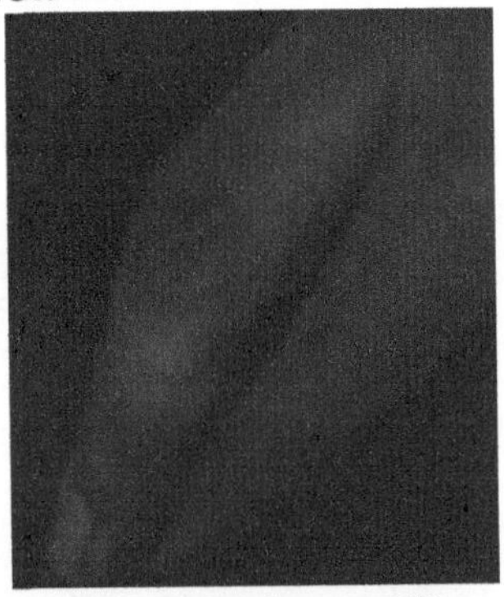

(See colour plate no. III)

Three fingers with middle finger tented

Palmar View

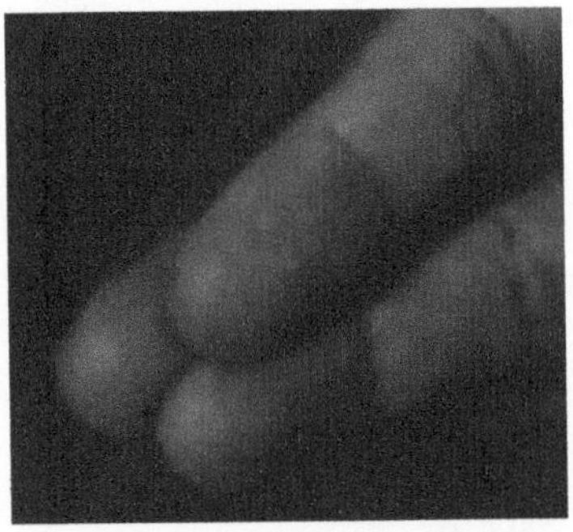

(See colour plate no. III)

Dorsal View

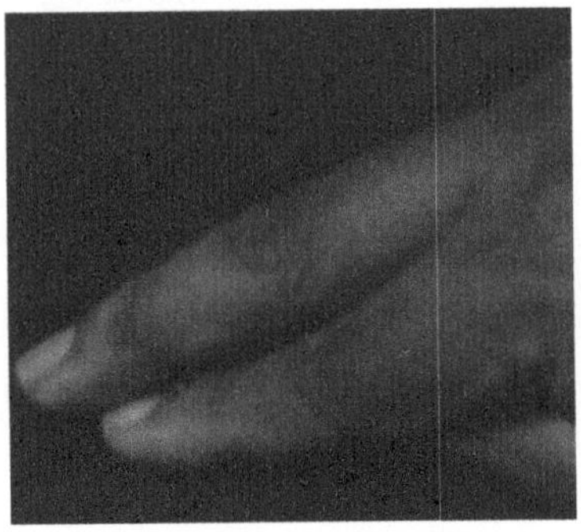

(See colour plate no. III)

Thenar or hypothenar surfaces of hand

Palmar View

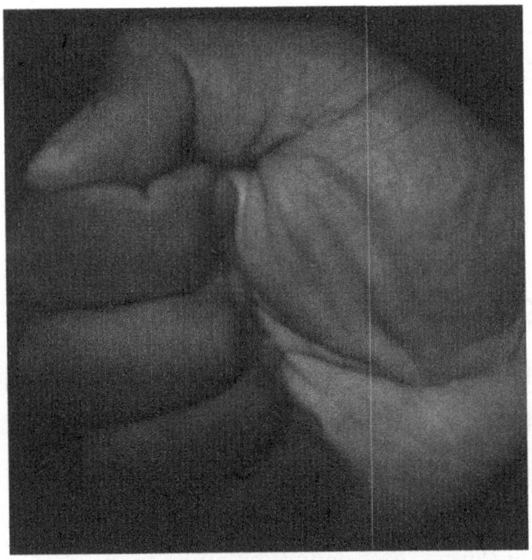

(See colour plate no. III)

MODIFICATIONS FOR PERCUSSIONS WITH DEVICES FOR NEONATE AND CHILDREN

1. **Paediatric anesthesia mask**

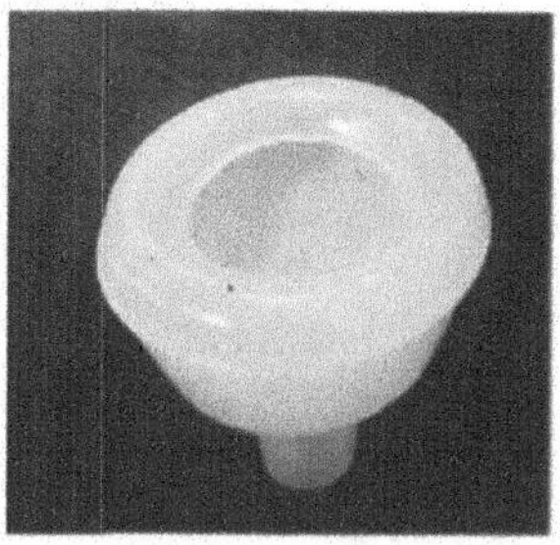

Hand placement using anaesthesia mask

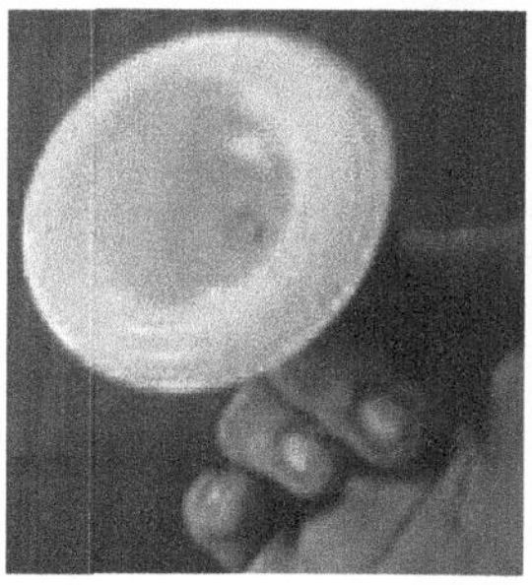

2. **Padded rubber nipples**

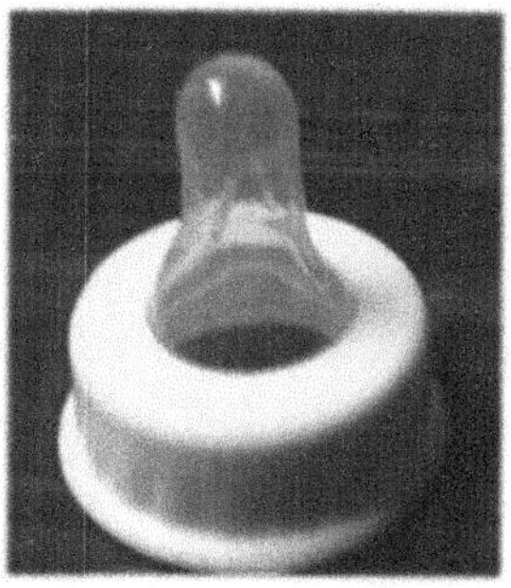

Hand placement using padded rubber nipples

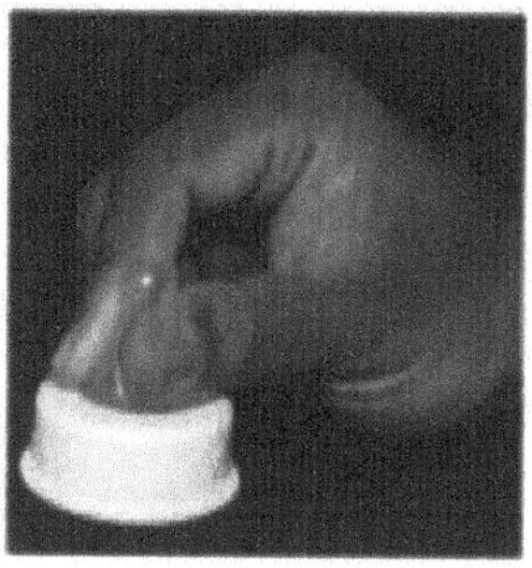

3. **Padded medicine cups large**

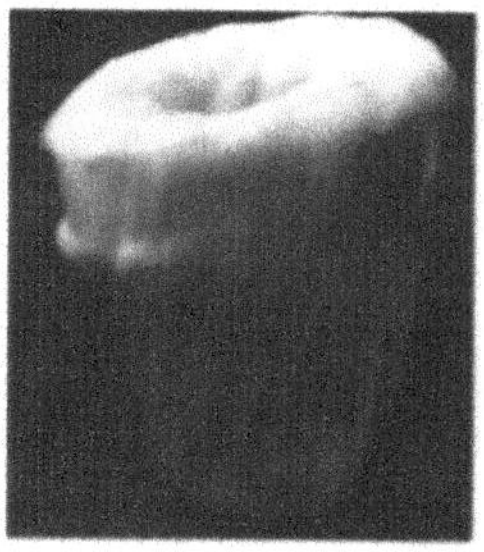

Hand placement using padded medicine cups large

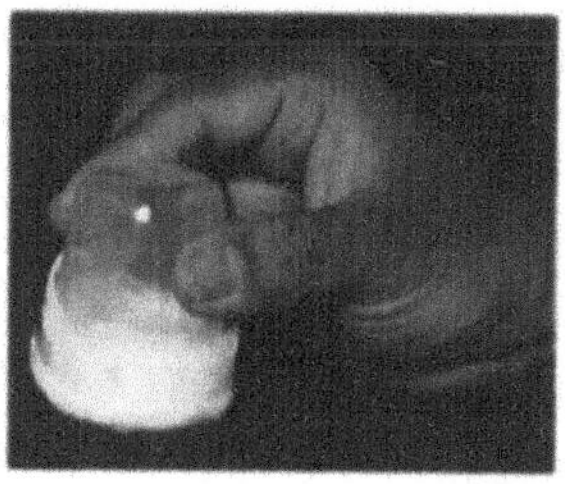

4. **Padded medicine cups small**

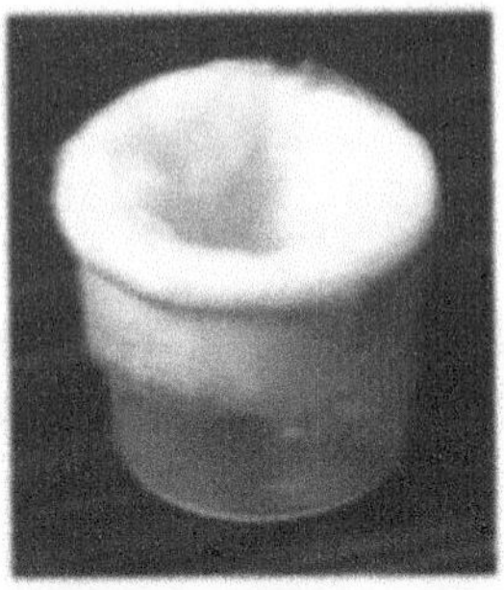

Hand placement using padded medicine cups small

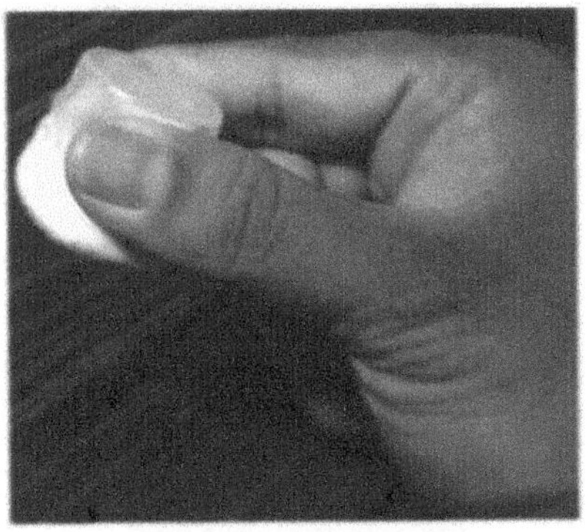

5. **Hand placement for percussion with Bell end of stethoscope**

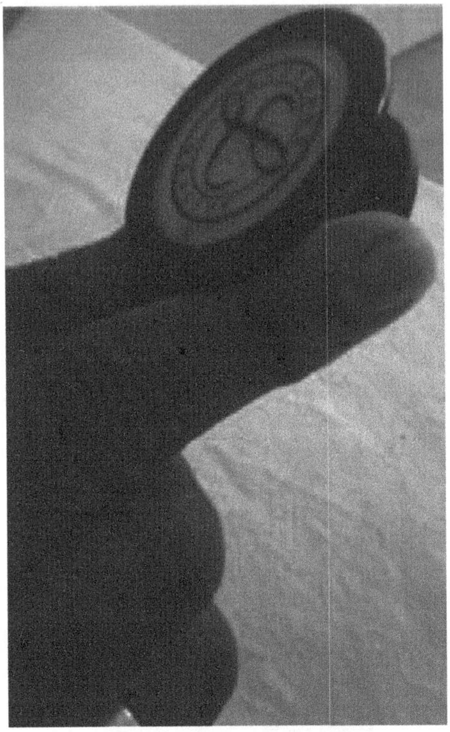

PARTS OF CENTRAL SUCTION APPARATUS

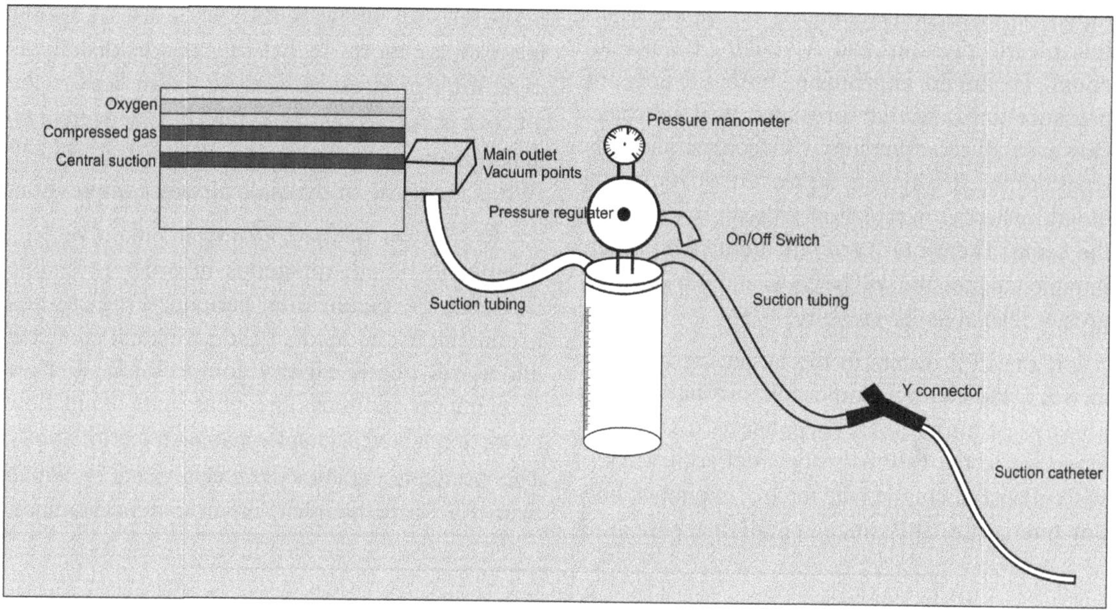

(See colour plate no. III)

EQUAL PRESSURE POINT

Equal pressure point (EPP) is the point where Intrapleural pressure and Alveolar pressure are equal. In forced expiration, both intrapleural pressure and alveolar pressure will increase. However, alveolar pressure will decrease along the length of the airway until a pressure of zero at the mouth, whereas intrapleural pressure will remain the same. Therefore there will be a point where intrapleural pressure will be equal and subsequently greater than alveolar pressure.

If the EPP occurs in the larger cartilaginous airways, the airway should collapse but still the airways remains open (because of cartilage). However, if the EPP is in the smaller airways, it will collapse. Increasing the force of expiration does not overcome EPP since it will increase both alveolar and intrapleural pressure. Another interesting concept is that EPP moves distally as expiration progresses because as air leaves the alveolar unit, the pressure in the alveolar decreases, hence the pressure in the airway decreases as well. EPP is the cause of dynamic airway compression.

Movement of the EPP toward the alveoli is thought to be advantageous in order to enable clearance of sputum from peripheral regions and to maximize the area of the bronchial tree that undergoes gentle airway compression, airflow acceleration and thus Two phase gas liquid flow exists (explained in chapter manual hyperinflation). This principle explains the mechanisms by which many ACTs are thought to effect sputum clearance.

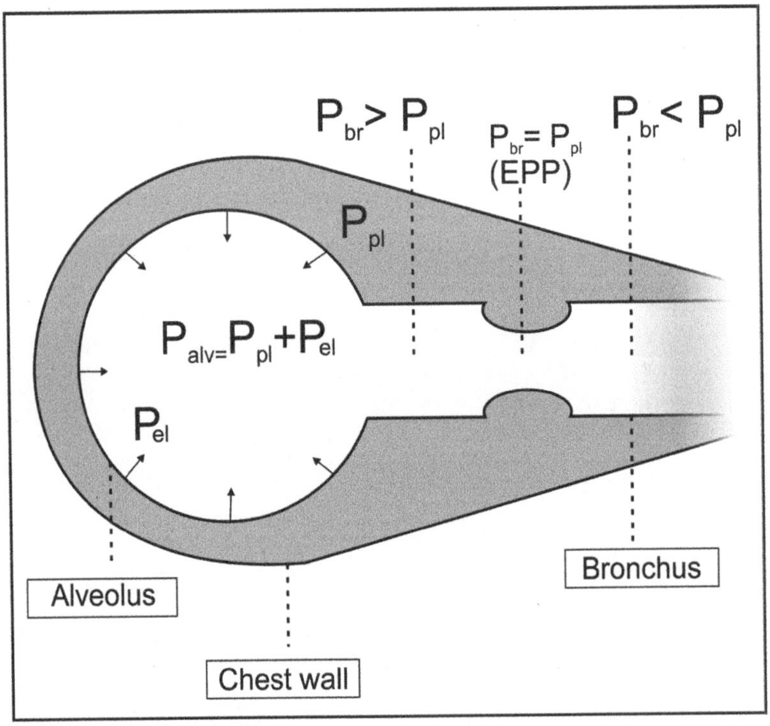

EPP: Equal pressure point; P_{alv}: Alveolar pressure; P_{br}: Bronchial pressure; P_{el}: Elastic recoil pressure; P_{pl}: Pleural pressure.

The EPP moves upstream (towards the alveoli) when the volume inside the lungs decreases and/or the pressure outside the airway increases. The EPP moves downstream (towards the mouth) when the volume inside the lungs increases and/or the pressure outside the airway decreases. Therefore, to move secretions from peripheral airways, it is more effective to commence huffing at low lung volumes and to progress to medium and finally large lung volumes.

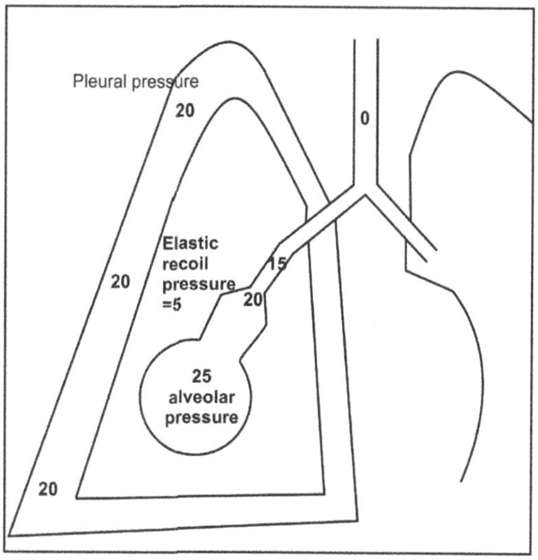

Figure shows static representation of dynamic state

Pleural pressure	=	+20 H_2O
Elastic recoil pressure	=	+5 cm
Pressure within alveoli	=	+25 cm

Macklem in 1974 located EPP are located in lobar or segmental bronchi at lung volume above FRC. Below FRC they progress towards alveoli.

There is a downward gradient from +25 to +20 to +15 and finally zero at the mouth. Somewhere along the airway the pressure within the airway will equal the pleural pressure to this which is called equal pressure point (20 cm in the above diagram). At this point dynamic collapse and compression of the airway takes place.

The dynamic collapse and compression of the airways during a forced expiratory manoeuvre is effective from points, choke points (Dawson and Elliott 1977), downstream of the equal pressure point. As the lung volume decreases these choke points move upstream (towards the alveoli) and at low lung volumes the more peripheral parts of the airways can be cleared. So a low huff shift EPP towards upstream or towards alveoli (more periphery) and a high huff shift EPP towards downstream or towards trachea (more towards central).

PARTS OF AMBUBAG

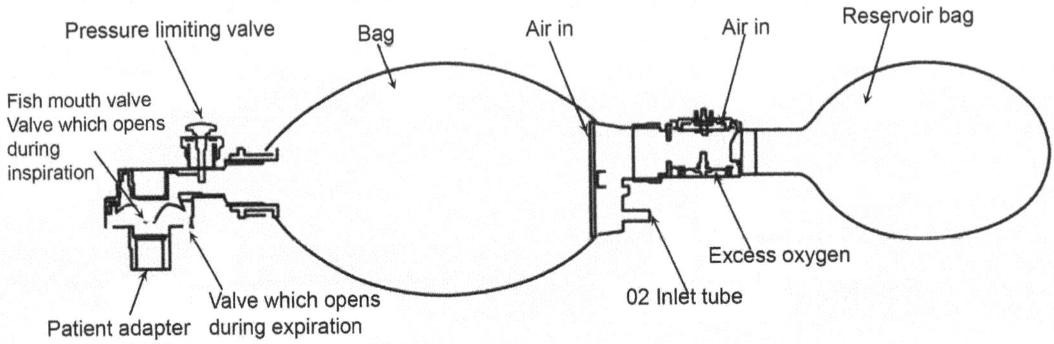

NEBULISER DELIVERY DEVIECS

Aerosol Drug Delivery System

Metered dose inhaler

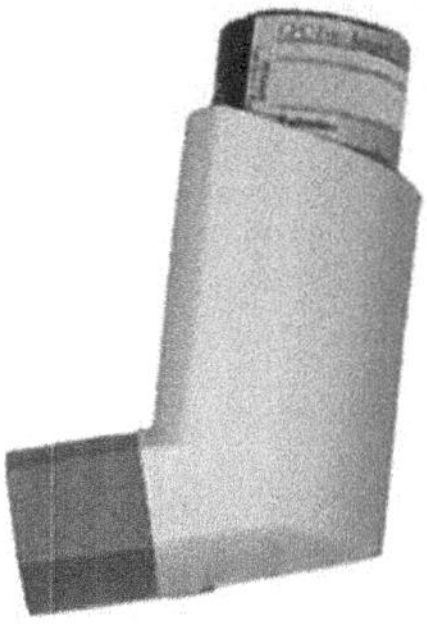

MDI Accessories: Spacer

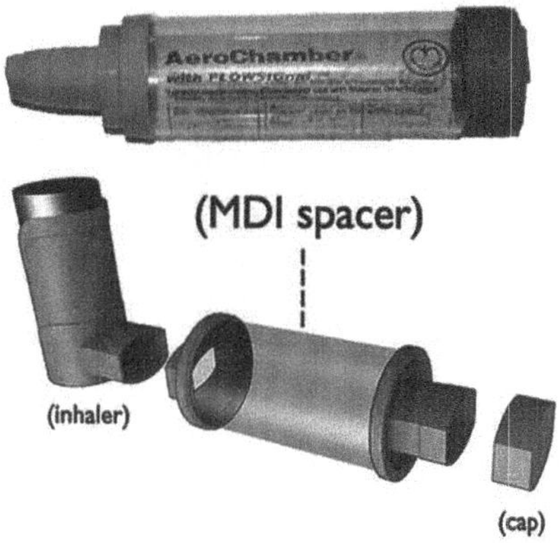

MDI accessories: Autohaler

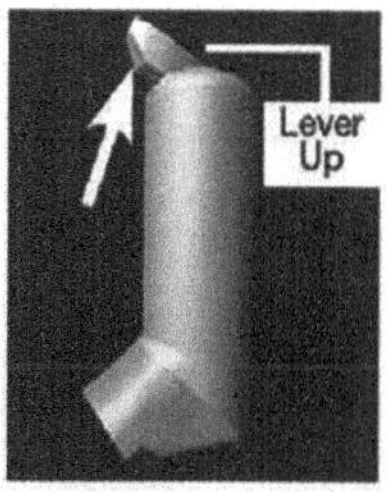

Dry powder inhaler: Rotahaler

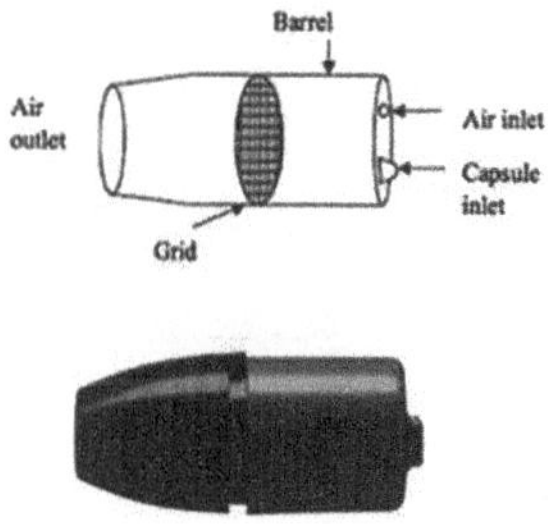

Dry powder inhaler: Spinhaler

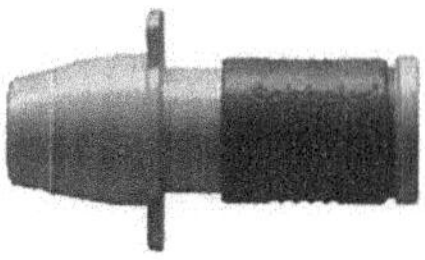

Dry powder inahler: Turbuhaler

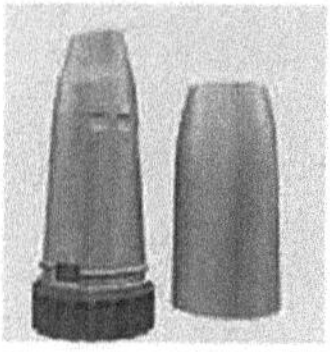

Hand bulb atomiser

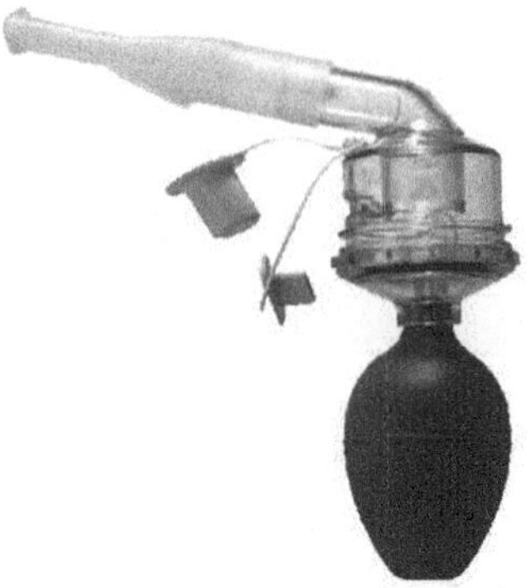

Large volume jet nebuliser

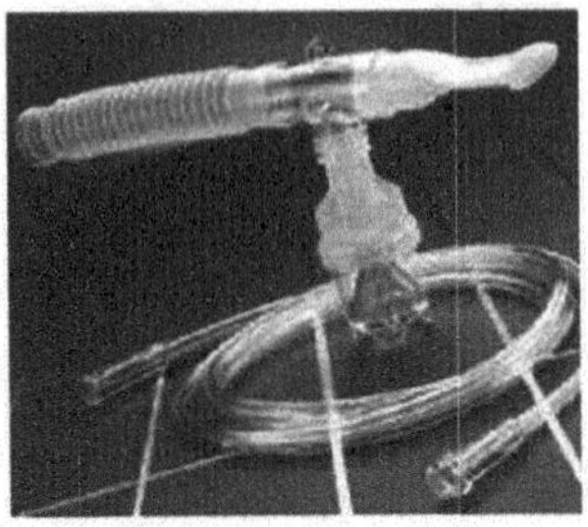

Small volume jet nebuliser

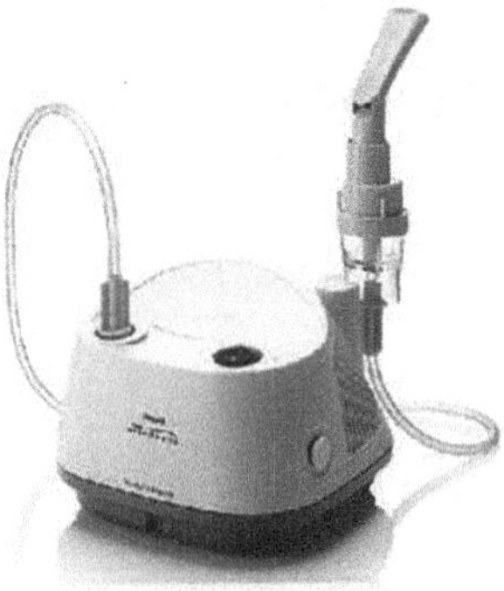

Ultrasonic nebuliser

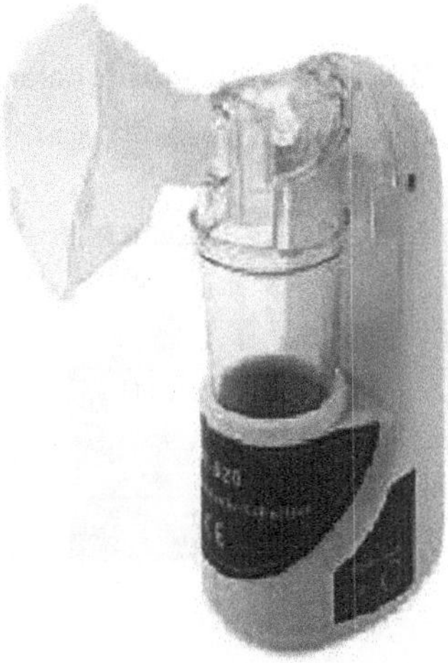

MANUAL THERAPY IN CARDIORESPIRATORY DISORDERS

1. Mobilisation for intervertebral joints (PA–Glide)

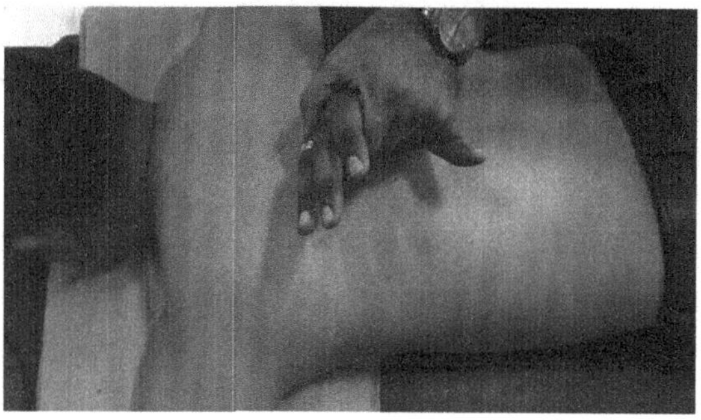

(See colour plate no. IV)

2. Superior glide of costotransverse joints

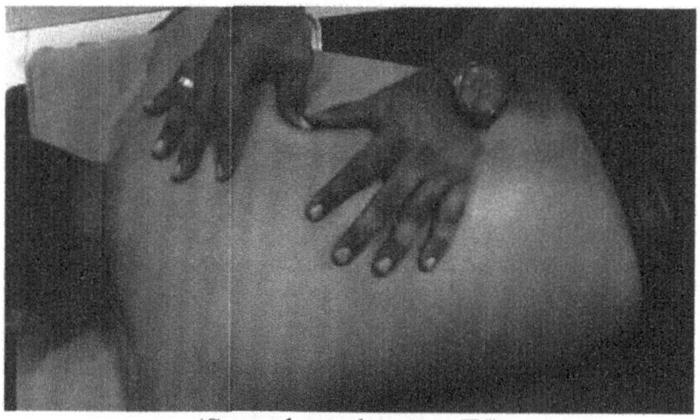

(See colour plate no. IV)

3. Inferior glide of costotransverse joint

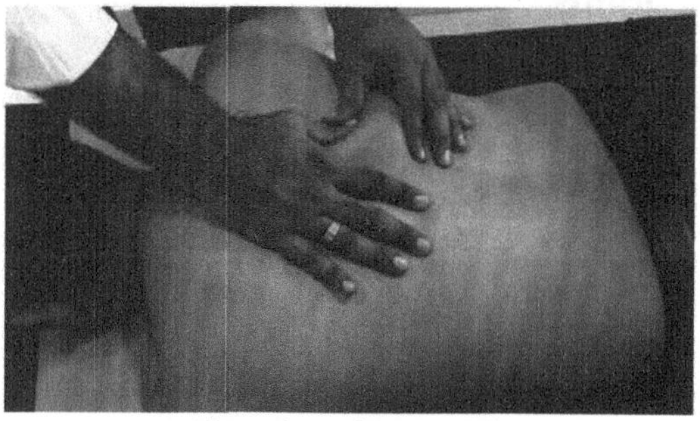

(See colour plate no. IV)

4A. Mobilisation of ribs in prone lying

Therapist applies pressure with thumbs superimposed each other in posteroanterior direction.

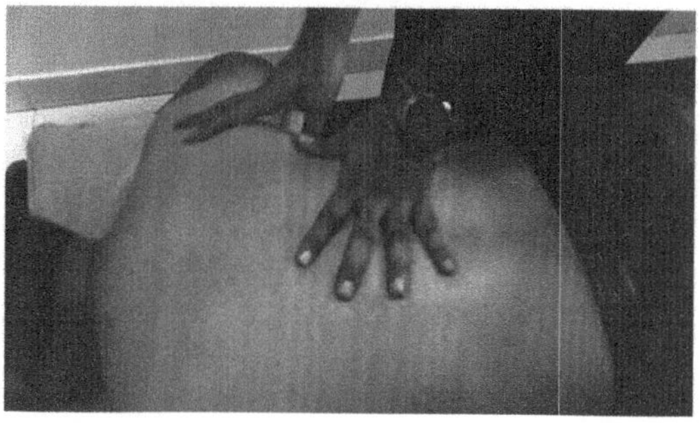

(See colour plate no. IV)

4B. Mobilisation of ribs in prone lying

In prone lying, one hand applies counter pressure, while the ulnar side of the mobilizing hand is positioned along the rib, from the rib angle.

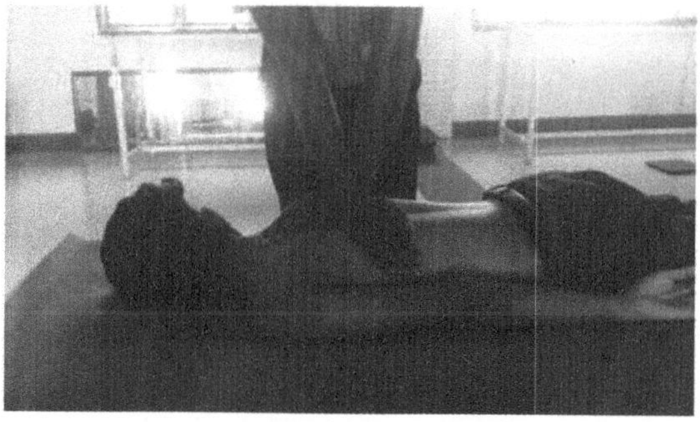

(See colour plate no. IV)

5. Mobilisation of ribs in supine lying

In supine lying patient places his both hands clasped under the neck, therapist places the hand underneath of patient thorax and pulls the ribs anteriorly.

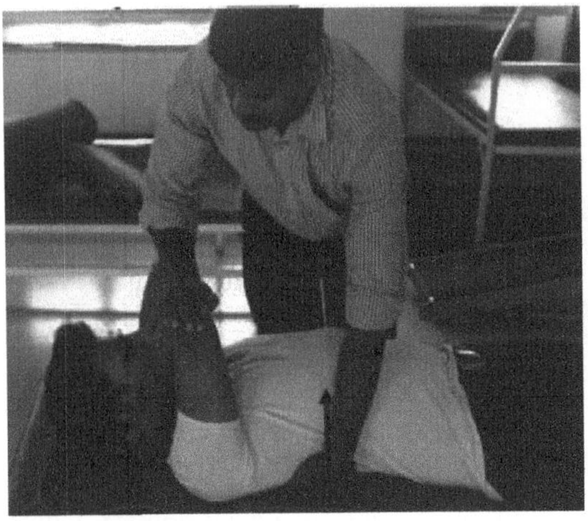

(See colour plate no. IV)

6. Aggressive mobilisation of ribs in modified supine lying

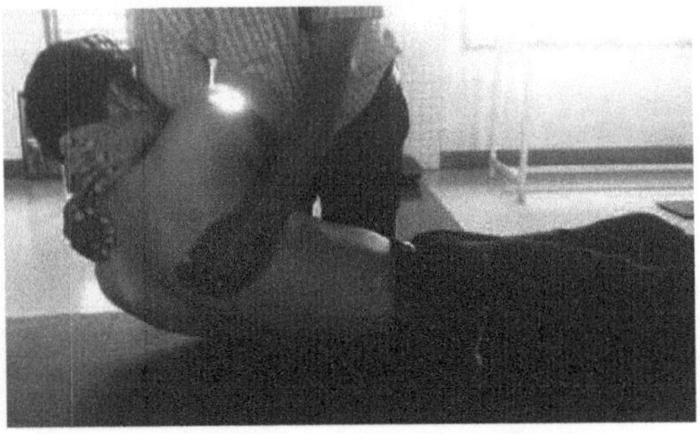

(See colour plate no. IV)

7. Mobilisation of facet joints

The patient is supine with his legs flexed and arms crossed in front of the chest. The operator rotates the patient passively toward himself and fixates the inferior vertebra of the involved segment with his thenar eminence and flexed middle finger over the transverse processes the index finger and thumb is positioned like a pistol grip and it is mobilised.

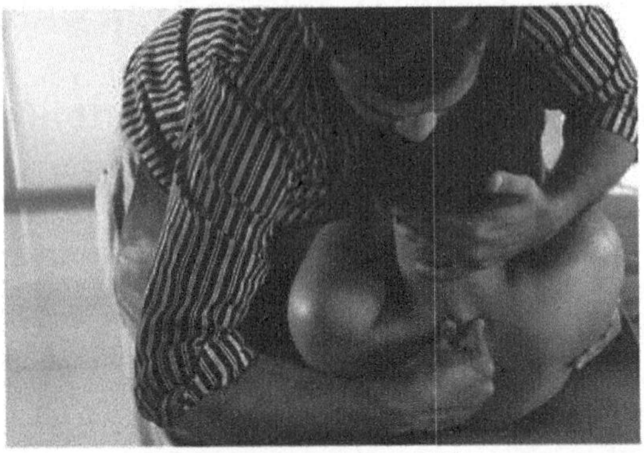

(See colour plate no. IV)

8. Mobilisation of facet joints with wedge

If therapist cannot hold the patient simultaneously while mobilising, a wedge can be used to create space for mobilising spinous processes.

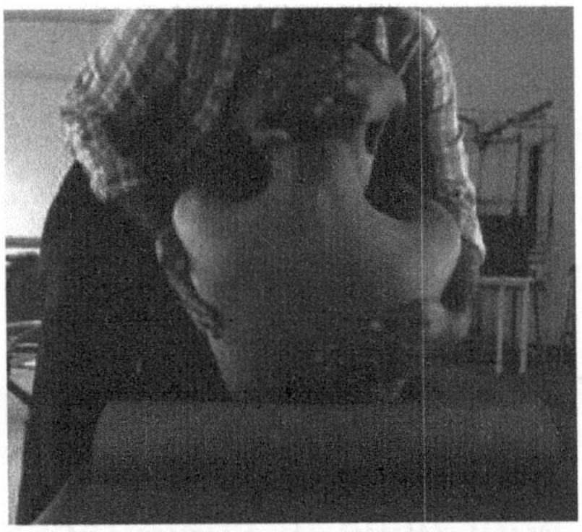

(See colour plate no. IV)

9. Mobilisation of costovertebral joints

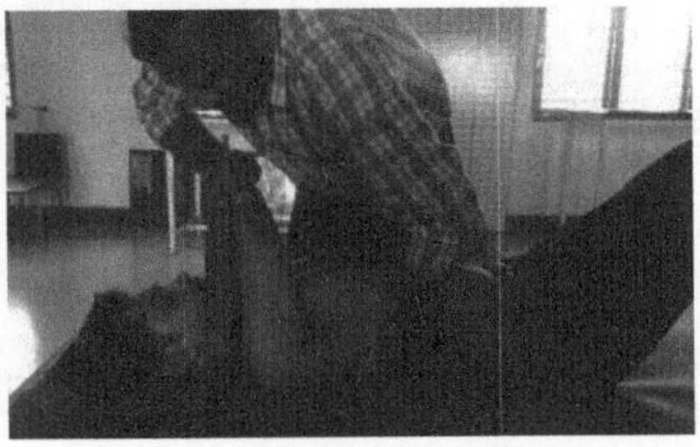

(See colour plate no. IV)

CHEST MOBILITY EXERCISES

1. To mobilise one side of the chest

Patient position: Sitting or standing

Starting position

Patient bends away from the tight side to lengthen tight structures and expand that side of the chest during inspiration. In the figure chest mobility exercise performed on the left side.

During inspiration patients bend towards the right side.

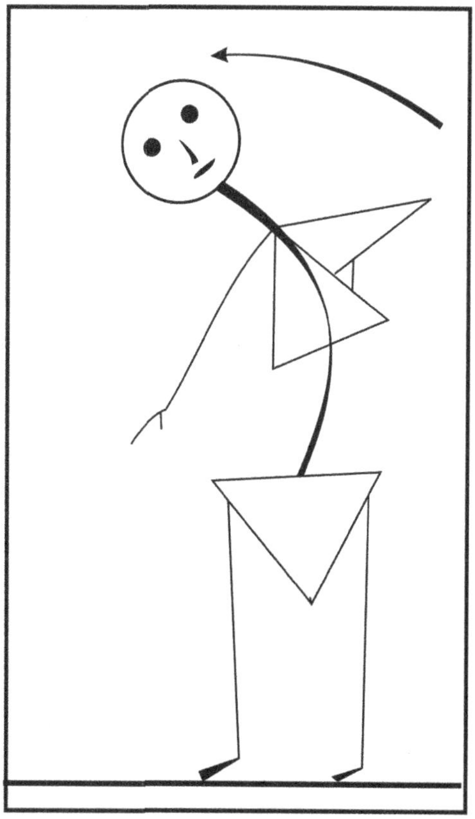

Ending position

The patient pushes the fisted hand into the lateral aspect of the chest, as he or she bends toward the tight side and breathes out during expiration.

During expiration patients bend towards the right side.

Progression

Patient raise the arm on the tight side of the chest over the head and side bend away from the tight side. This will place an additional stretch on the tight tissues.

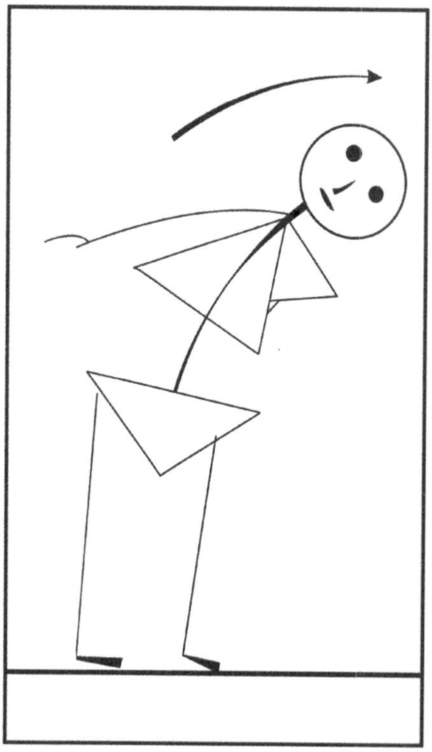

2. To mobilise the upper chest and stretch the pectoralis muscles

Patient position: Sitting position

Starting position

Patient is sitting in a chair (without arm rest) with hands clasped behind the head, have him or her horizontally abduct the arms (elongating the pectoralis muscles) during a deep inspiration (extension of thorax and neck has to be performed).

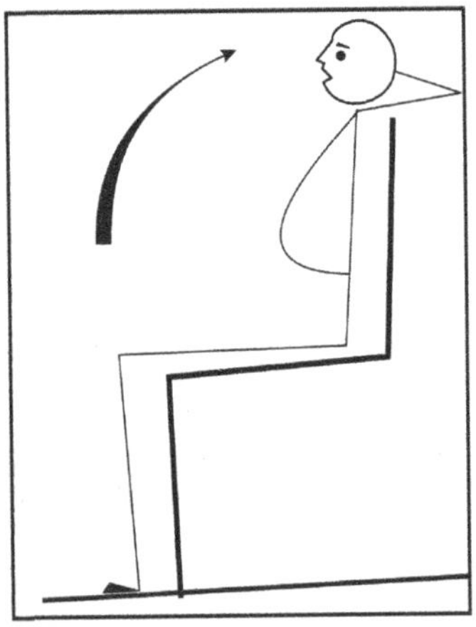

Ending position

Then, instruct the patient to bring the elbows together and bend forward during expiration.

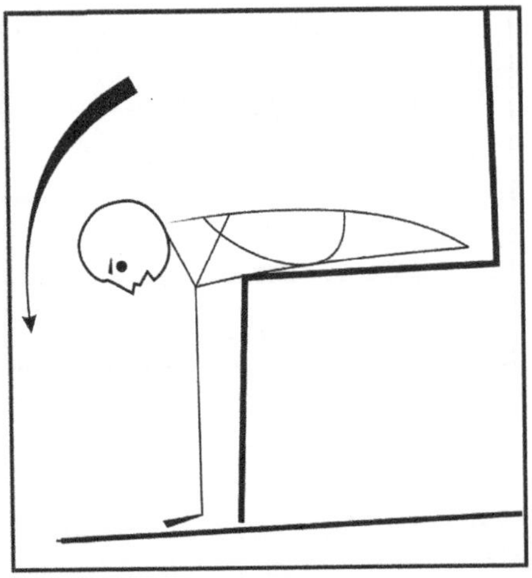

3. To mobilise the upper chest and shoulders

Patient position: Sitting position

Starting position

With the patient sitting in a chair, have him or her reach with both arms overhead (180 degrees bilateral shoulder flexion and slight abduction) during inspiration (with neck and trunk extension).

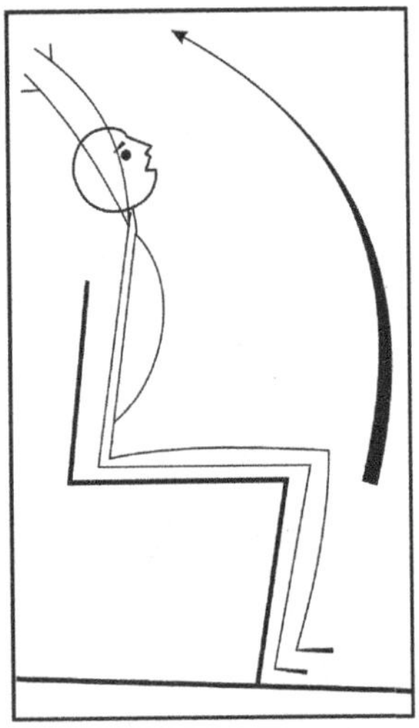

Ending position

Then have the patient bend forward at the hips and reach for the floor during expiration (with neck and trunk flexion).

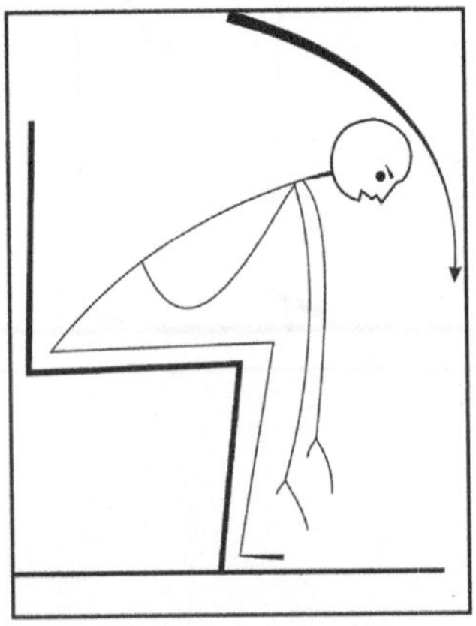

Patient position: Standing position

Starting position

With the patient sitting in a chair, have him or her reach with both arms overhead (180 degrees bilateral shoulder flexion and slight abduction) during inspiration (with neck and trunk hyperextension).

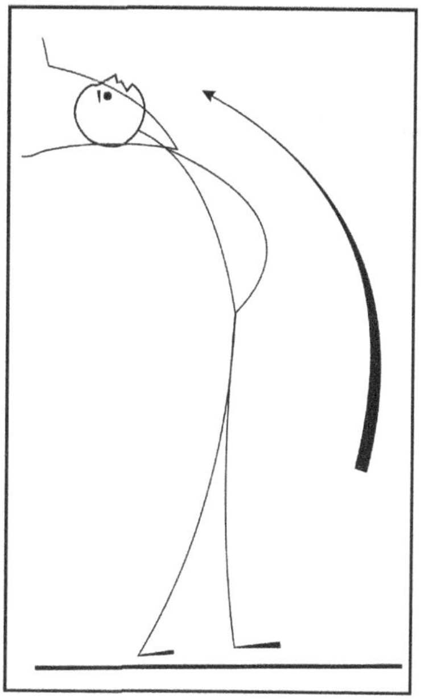

Ending position

Then have the patient bend forward at the hips and reach for the floor during expiration (with neck and trunk flexion).

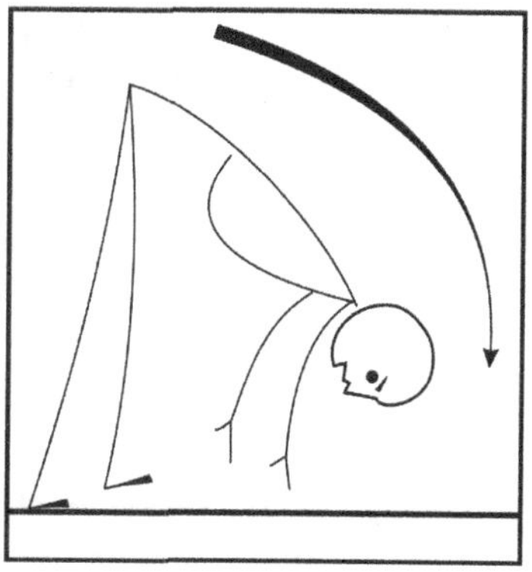

4. To increase expiration during deep breathing

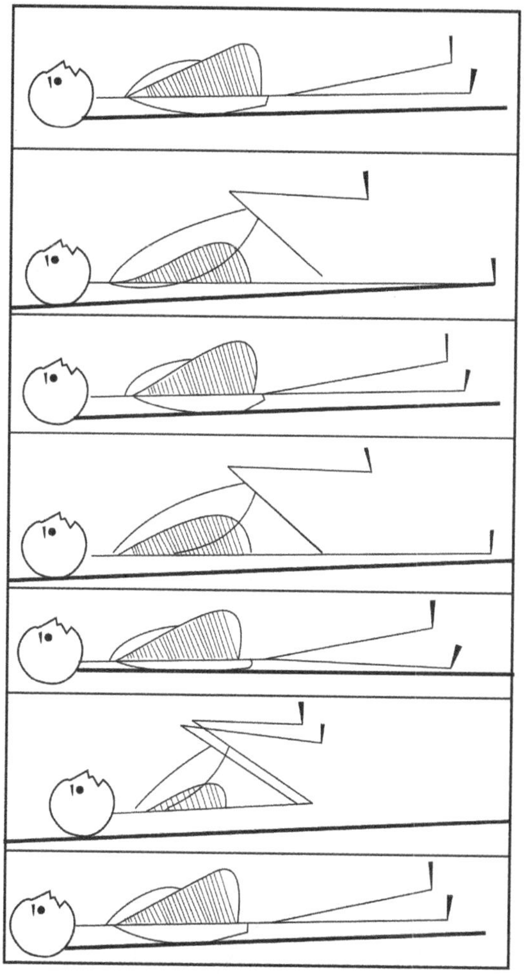

Patient position: Supine lying

Patient breathe in while in a hook-lying position (hips and knees are slightly flexed). Then, instruct the patient to pull one knees to the chest during expiration.

Again patient make the knee extended with inspiration. Then instruct the patient to pull the other knee to the chest during expiration.

Again patient make the knee extended with inspiration.

Finally both knees are pulled towards the chest during expiration. (Please note knee flexion is coordinated with expiration and knee extension is coordinated with inspiration).

5. Wand Exercises

a. Shoulder flexion and abduction

Starting position: Standing

Equipment required: Wand (Stick)

Patient should be in standing grasping the wand with both hands a shoulder width apart and lifting the stick overhead. Patient should coordinate shoulders flexion during inspiration and shoulder extension during expiration.

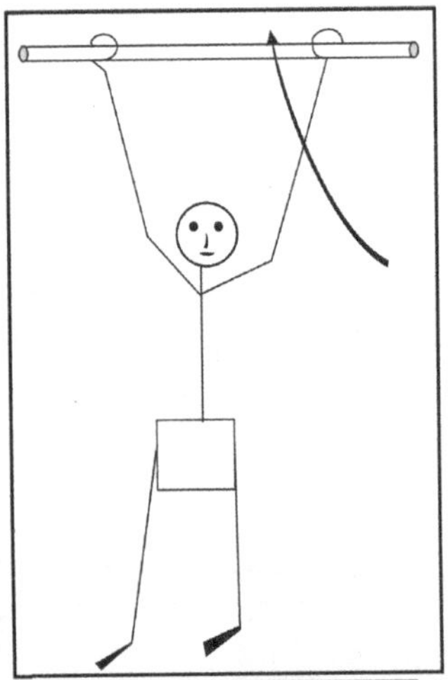

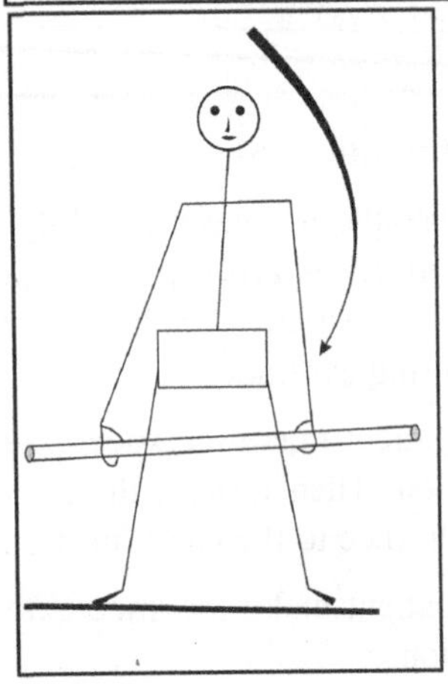

b. Shoulder external and internal rotation

In starting position, patient in standing, the patients shoulder are abducted 90 degrees and in internal rotation and the elbow are flexed 90 degrees. Wand is grasped by both hands. During inspiration patient will perform external rotation, the wand is moved towards patients head. During expiration the patient will perform internal rotation; the wand is moved towards waist line.

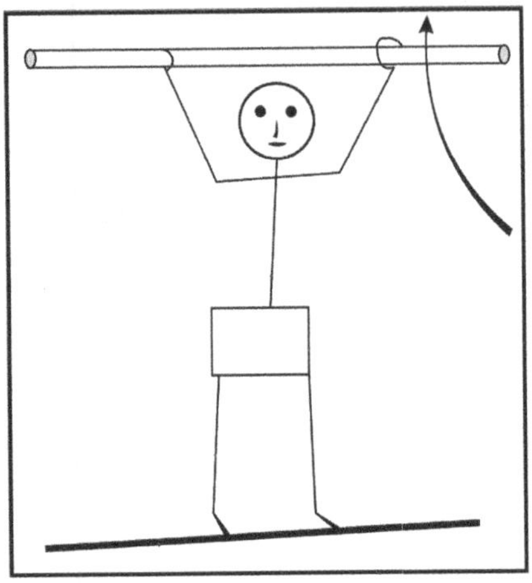

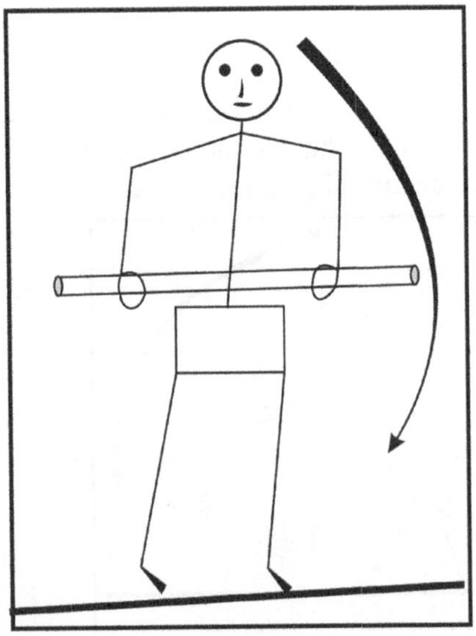

BELT EXERCISES

Unilateral posterior basal expansion exercises

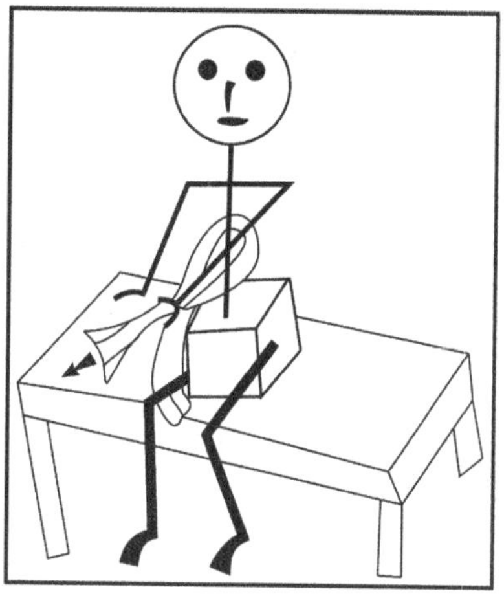

Equipment required: Rolled bed sheet

Patient in high sitting

Bed sheet has to be rolled. The one end of the bed sheet is placed under the opposite side thigh. The towel is rolled back and placed along the posterior thorax. The other end is kept in the patients hand on the side where expansion has to be given. Patient will pull the rolled bed sheet in the forward direction (see arrow mark in the figure) during expiration. During inspiration patient has to release the bed sheet slowly.

Unilateral lateral basal expansion exercises

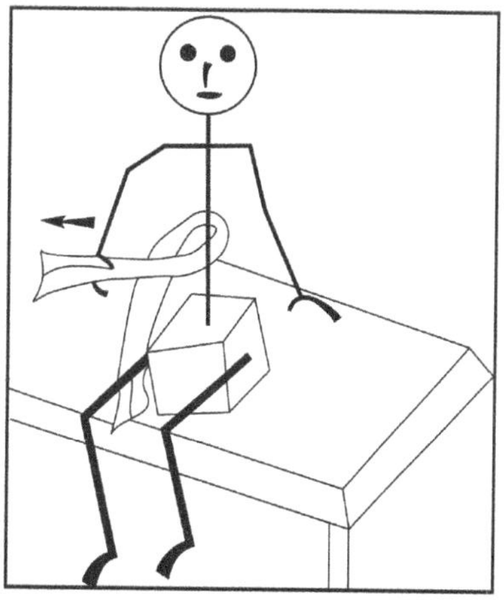

Equipment required: Rolled bed sheet

Patient in high sitting

Bed sheet has to be rolled. The one end of the bed sheet is placed under the opposite side thigh. The towel is rolled back and placed along the posterior thorax. The other end is kept in the patients hand on the opposite side where expansion has to be given. Patient will pull the rolled bed sheet towards the opposite side (see arrow mark in the figure) during expiration. During inspiration patient has to release the bed sheet slowly.

Bilateral lateral basal expansion exercises

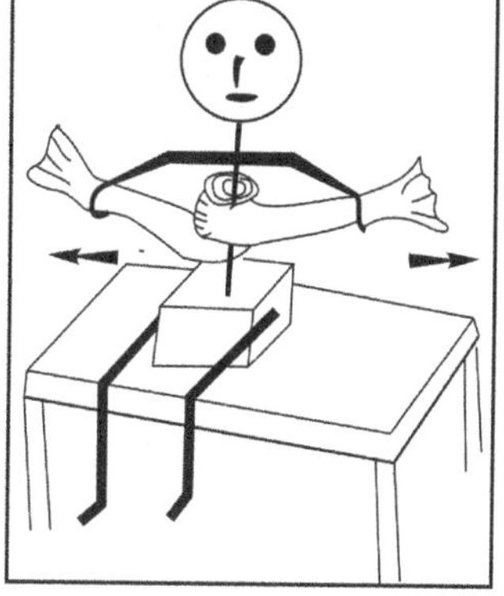

Equipment required: Rolled bed sheet

Patient in high sitting

Bed sheet has to be rolled. The towel is rolled back and placed along the posterior thorax. Both end of the sheet placed in the opposite hands. Patient will pull the rolled bed sheet ends each other (see arrow mark in the figure) during expiration. During inspiration patient has to release the bed sheet slowly.

ELECTRODE PLACEMENT OF TENS IN ABDOMINAL INCISIONS

(A) Vertical incisions

Type of TENS: Intense TENS

Electrode placement: On either side of the incision.

Description: High intensity high frequency TENS.

(B) Oblique or transverse incisions (even also in Thoracotomy)

Type of TENS: Intense TENS

Electrode placement: Above the incision site

Description: High intensity high frequency TENS.

(A)

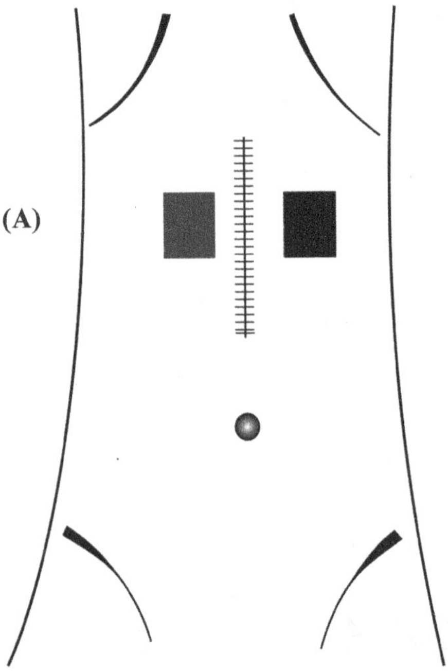

(B)

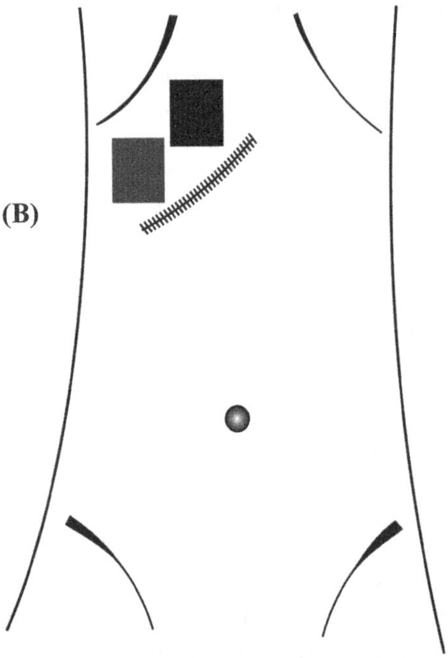

References

1. Francois Haas. Pulmonary therapy and Rehabilitation. Williams and Wilkins, Baltimore, 1991.
2. Alvarez SE, Peterson M, Lunsford BR. Respiratory treatment of the adult patient with spinal cord injury. Physical Therapy 1981:61(12):1737-1745.
3. B Vyas, S Shah, H Tiwari, A Singh. The effect of Acu-TENS on FEV1, six-minute walk distance and dyspnoea in patients with chronic obstructive pulmonary disease: A randomised trial. International Journal of Biomedical and Advance Research 2013; 4(7): 448-454.
4. Barbara A, Webber and Jennifer, A Pryor. Physiotherapy for Respiratory and Cardiac Problems, Edinburgh, London, Madrid, Melbourne, Newyork, 1993.
5. Bott J, Blumenthal S, Buxton M, Ellum S, Falconer C, Garrod R *et al.* Guidelines for the physiotherapy management of the adult, medical, spontaneously breathing patient. Thorax 2009; 64(Suppl 1):i1-i52.
6. Bourjeily-Habr G, Rochester CL, Palermo F, *et al.* Randomised controlled trial of transcutaneous electrical muscle stimulation of the lower extremities in patients with chronic obstructive pulmonary disease. Thorax 2002; 57:1045-49.
7. Cahalin L, Braga M, Matsuo Y, Hernandez E. Efficacy of Diaphragmatic Breathing in Persons with Chronic Obstructive Pulmonary Disease: A Review of the Literature. Journal of Cardiopulmonary Rehabilitation 2002; 22(1):7-21.
8. Claudia R, Levenson. Breathing exercises: In Cynthia Coffin Zadai. Pulmonary Management in Physical Therapy. 1st ed. NY (USA): Churchill Livingstone Inc., 1992.
9. Derenne J, Macklem PT, Roussos CH. The Respiratory muscles: Mechanics, Control and Pathophysiology, Part I, Am Rev Respir Dis 1978; 118:119-133.
10. Donna L Frownfelter. Chest Physical Therapy and Pulmonary Rehabilitation–An Interdisciplinary Approach. 2nd ed., St. Louis (USA): Mosby Year Book Medical Publisher 1987; 233.
11. Donrawee Leelarungrayub chapter 20 Chest Mobilization Techniques for Improving Ventilation and Gas Exchange in Chronic Lung Disease Chapter from the book Chronic Obstructive Pulmonary Disease – Current Concepts and Practice. Available from URL: www.intechopen.com .http://www.intechopen.com/books/chronic-obstructivepulmonary-disease-current-concepts-and-practice.
12. Hough A. Physiotherapy in respiratory care. Cheltenham: Nelson Thornes, 2001.
13. Irwin S, Tecklin J. Cardiopulmonary physical therapy. St. Louis, Mo.: Mosby, 2004.
14. Joanne Watchie. Cardiopulmonary Physical Therapy, WB Saunders, Philadelphia, 1995.
15. John R Bach. Pulmonary Rehabilitation. Hanley and Belfus, Philadelphia, 1995.
16. Kang SW. Pulmonary rehabilitation in patients with neuromascular disease. Yonsei Med J 2006; 47(3):307-314.
17. Ken SL Laul, Alice YM Jones. A single session of Acu-TENS increases FEV1 and reduces dyspnoea in patients with chronic obstructive pulmonary disease: A randomised, placebo-controlled trial Australian Journal of Physiotherapy 2008; 54: 179-184.
18. Kisner C, Colby L. Therapeutic exercise. Philadelphia: F.A. Davis, 1996.
19. Marc Roig, Reid WD. Electrical stimulation and peripheral muscle function in COPD: A systematic review Respiratory Medicine 2009;103:485-495.

20. Mila Diamond. Lose weight by breathing…Really! Beautiful confident you! 2012. Available from URL: http:/ /www.womensperfectbody.com/fatloss/lose-weight-by-proper-breathing.
21. Montero JC, Feldman DJ, Montero D. Effects of Glossopharyngeal breathing on respiratory function after cervical cord transaction. Arch Phys Med rehabil 1967;48(12): 650-653.
22. Mounika. 6 Yoga breathing techniques for weight loss. Stylecraze. com. 2014. Available from URL: http:// www.stylecraze.com/articles/6-yoga-breathingtechniques-for-weight-loss.
23. Moyna J Parker, Physiotherapy in Thoracic Conditions. Lecture Notes, University of Alberta, 1984.
24. Patrica A Downie, Textbook of Heart, Chest Vascular Disease for physiotherapists, JP Bros.
25. Paula Agostini, Sally Singh. Incentive spirometry following thoracic surgery: What should we be doing? Physiotherapy 2009; 95:76–82.
26. Pryor J, Webber B. International Perspectives in Physical therapy. Respiratory care. Singapore: Churchill Livingstone, 1991.
27. Roussos CS, Fixley M, Genest J *et al.* Voluntary factors influencing the distribution of Inspired gas, Am Rev Respir Dis 1977;116:457.
28. Scanlan C, Spearman C, Sheldon R, Egan D. Egan's fundamentals of respiratory care. St. Louis: Mosby, 1990.
29. Thomas Ahrens, Marin Kollef, Jena Stewart, William Shannon. Effect of kinetic therapy on Pulmonary complications Am J Crit Care 2004;13: 376-382.
30. Vibekk P (1991) Chest mobilization and respiratory function, In: Respiratory care, Pryor JA (Ed). 103-119, Churchill Livingstone. ISBN 0-443-03611, Tokyo.
31. Vivodtzev I, Lacasse Y, Maltais F. Neuromuscular electrical stimulation of the lower limbs in patients with chronic obstructive pulmonary disease J Cardiopul Rehab Prev 2008; 28:79-91.
32. Vivodtzev I, Pe´pin JL, Vottero G, *et al.* Improvements in quadriceps strength and dyspnea in daily tasks after 1 month of electrical stimulation in severely deconditioned and malnourished COPD. Chest 2006; 129: 1540-48.
33. Warren VC. Glossopharyngeal and neck accessory muscle breathing in a young adult with C2 complete tetraplegia resulting in ventilator dependency. Phys. Ther 2001; 82(6):590-600.
34. Wetzel JL. Management of respiratory dysfunction. In: Edelle C. field, Editor. Spinal cord Injury rehabilitation FA Davis 2009; 337-392.
35. Wuyam B, Borel JC, Vivodtzev I. The role of non-invasive measurement of ventilation during exercise, electrostimulation of the quadriceps, and the work of breathing in the rehabilitation of patients with chronic obstructive pulmonary disease Rev Mal Respir 2005; 22 (7s):76-78.
36. Zanotti E, Felicetti G, Maini M, *et al.* Peripheral muscle strength training in bed-bound patients with COPD receiving mechanical ventilation: Effect of electrical stimulation. Chest 2003;124: 292-96.
37. Rodrigues J. and Watchie J (2010). Cardiovascular and pulmonary physical therapy treatment, In: Cardiovascular and pulmonary physical therapy–A clinical Manual.
38. Watchie J (Ed), 2nd edition, 319-322, Saunders, ISBN 978-0-7216-0646-0, Missouri.
39. American Thoracic Society/European Respiratory Society Statement on Pulmonary Rehabilitation (2006). American journal of respiratory and critical care medicine, Vol.170, 1390-1413, ISSN 1535-4970.
40. Cane LD (1992). Functional anatomy and physiology of ventilation In: Pulmonary management in physical therapy. Zadai CC, (Ed), Churchill Livingstone, 13-18, ISBN 0443087415, Tokyo.
41. Celli BR (2000). Exercise in the rehabilitation of patients with respiratory disease, In: Pulmonary rehabilitation. Guideline to success, Hodgkin JE, Celli BR, Connors GL (Eds). Lippincott, Williams and Wilkins 156-157. ISBN 9780781719896, Philadelphia.

42. Frownfelter D (1987). Chest Physical therapy and pulmonary rehabilitation, 2nd edition, 170-177, Year book medical publishers, ISBN 0-8151-3340-5, Chicago.

43. Grant R (2001). Physical therapy of the cervical and thoracic spine, 3rd edition, Churchill Livingstone, 45-60, ISBN 0-443-07155-1, New York.

44. Greenman, P (1996). Principles of manual medicine, 2nd edition, Williams and Wilkins, ISBN 0683035584, Baltimore.

45. Jennifer A and Prasad SA (2008). Physiotherapy techniques, In: Physiotherapy for respiratory and cardiac problems, 4th ed, Pryor JA, Prasad SA (Eds), 188-190, Churchill Livingstone, ISBN 9780080449852, Toronto.

46. Kisner C and Colby LA (1996). Therapeutic exercise: Foundations and technique, 3rd edition, FA Davis Company, 143-182, ISBN 0-683-04576-8, Philadelphia.

47. Reid WD and Chung F (2004). Chest radiology In: Clinical management notes and case histories in Cardiopulmonary physical therapy 31-36. Slack Incoporated, ISBN 1-55642-568-6, New Jersey.

48. Wetzel JL, Lunsford BR, Peterson MJ and Alvarez SE (1995). Respiratory Rehabilitation of the patients with a spinal cord injury, In: Cardiopulmonary rehabilitation, 3rd ed, Irwin S, Tecklin JS (Eds), 596, Mosby, ISBN 0-8016-7926-5, Wiesbaden.

49. Subin Rao V, Prem V, Sahoo. Effect of upper limb, lower limb and combined training on health-related quality of life in COPD. Lung India [serial online] 2010 [cited 2017 Sep 20];27:4-7. Available from: http://www.lungindia.com/text.asp?2010/27/1/4/59260.

50. Carter R, Holiday DB, Stocks J, Tiep B. Peak physiologic responses to arm and leg ergometry in male and female patients with Air flow obstruction. Chest 2003;124:511-18.

51. Holland AE, Hill CJ, Nehez E, Ntoumenopoulos G. Does unsupported upper limb exercise training improve symptoms and quality of life for patients with chronic obstructive pulmonary disease? J Cardiopulm Rehabil 2004;24:422-27.

52. Ries AL, Ellis B Hawkins RW. Upper extremity exercise training in chronic obstructive pulmonary disease. Chest 1988;82:688-92.

53. Martinez FJ, Voget PD, Dupont DN, Beamis JF, Stanoponlos I. Supported arm exercise vs unsupported arm exercise in rehabilitation of patients with chronic airflow obstruction. Chest 1993;103:1397-402.

54. Lake FR, Kathrun H, Tom B, Shaw JO, Musk W. Upper limb and lower limb exercise training in patients with chronic airflow obstruction. Chest 1990;97;1077-82.

55. Takahashi T, Jenkins SC, Geoffrey RS, Carol PW, Lake FR. A new unsupported upper limb exercise test for patients with chronic obstructive pulmonary disease. J Cardiol Pulm Rehabil 2003;23:430-37.

56. Arm training reduces VO 2 and VE cost of unsupported arm exercise and elevation in chronic obstructive pulmonary disease. J Cardiopulm Rehabil 1997;17:171-77.

57. Velloso M, Stella GS, Cendon S. Metabolic and ventilatory parameters of four activities of daily living accomplished with arms in COPD patients. Chest 2003;123:1047-53.

58. Subin Solomen, Pravin Aaron International Journal of Physical Education, Sports and Health 2015; 2(2): 237-241.

59. Subin Solomen, Komal Agarwal Comparative study between chest mobility exercises with incentive spirometry versus chest mobility exercises with stacked breathing on chest expansion in subjects with unilateral pleural effusion International Journal of Development Research 2016; 06:8034-8038.

60. Postural drainage therapy AARC practice guideline: Respir. Care 1991;36(12):1418-1426.

61. Incentive Spirometry. AARC Clinical Practice Guideline Respir Care 1991;36(12):1402–05.

62. Endotracheal suctioning of mechanically ventilated patients with artificial airways AARC Clinical Practice Guidelines. Respir Care 2010 Jun;55(6):758-64.
63. L Denehy. The use of manual hyperinflation in airway clearance European Respiratory Journal 1999 14: 958-65.
64. Barker M, Adams S. An evaluation of a single chest physiotherapy treatment on mechanically ventilated patients with acute lung injury Physiotherapy Research International 7 (2002), 157-69.
65. Berney S, Denehy L. A comparison of the effects of manual and ventilator hyperinflation on static lung compliance and sputum production in intubated and ventilated intensive care patients Physiotherapy Research International 7 (2002), 100-08.
66. Clapham L, Harrison J, Raybould T. A multidisciplinary audit of manual hyperinflation technique (sigh breath) in a neurosurgical intensive care unit Intensive and Critical Care Nursing 11 (1995), 265-71.
67. Clarke RC, Kelly BE, Convery PN, Fee JP. Ventilatory characteristics in mechanically ventilated patients during manual hyperventilation for chest physiotherapy Anaesthesia 54 (1999), 936-40.
68. Clement AJ, Hübsch SK. Chest physiotherapy by the bag squeezing method: A guide to technique Physiotherapy 54 (1968), 355-59.
69. Hila J, Ellis E, Holmes W. Feedback withdrawal and changing compliance during manual hyperinflation Physiotherapy Research International 7 (2002), 53-64.
70. Hodgson C, Carroll S, Denehy L. A survey of manual hyperinflation in Australian hospitals Australian Journal of Physiotherapy 45 (1999), 185-93.
71. Jellema WT, Groeneveld AB, van Goudoever J, Wesseling KH, Westerhof N, Lubbers MJ, Kesecioglu J, Van Lieshout JJ. Hemodynamic effects of intermittent manual lung hyperinflation in patients with septic shock Heart and Lung 29 (2000), 356-66.
72. Jones AYM, Hutchinson RC, Lin E, Oh TE. Peak expiratory flow rates produced with the Laerdal and Mapleson-C bagging circuits Australian Journal of Physiotherapy 38 (1992), 211-215.
73. Jones AYM, Hutchinson RC, Oh TE. Chest physiotherapy practice in intensive care units in Australia, the UK and Hong Kong Physiotherapy Theory and Practice 8 (1992), 39-47.
74. Jones AYM, Jones RD, Bacon-Shone J. A comparison of expiratory flow rates in two breathing circuits used for manual inflation of the lungs Physiotherapy 77 (1991), 593-97.
75. Maxwell L, Crosbie J Ellis E. A new system for examining pattern of ventilation Australian Journal of Physiotherapy 47 (2001), 271.
76. Maxwell LJ, Ellis ER. The effects of three manual hyperinflation techniques on pattern of ventilation in a test lung model Anaesthesia and Intensive Care 30 (2002), 283-88.
77. Maxwell LJ, Ellis ER. The effect of circuit type, volume delivered and "rapid release" on flow rates during manual hyperinflation Australian Journal of Physiotherapy 49 (2003), 31-38.
78. McCarren B, Chow CM. Manual hyperinflation: A description of the technique, Australian Journal of Physiotherapy 42 (1996), 203-08.
79. Ntoumenopoulos G, Gild A, Cooper DJ. The effect of manual lung hyperinflation and postural drainage on pulmonary complications in mechanically ventilated trauma patients Anaesthesia and Intensive Care 26 (1998), 492-96.

80. Paratz J, Lipman J, McAuliffe M. Effect of manual hyperinflation on hemodynamics, gas exchange, and respiratory mechanics in ventilated patients Journal of Intensive Care Medicine 17 (2002), 317-24.

81. Patman S, Jenkins S, Bostock S, Edlin S. Cardiovascular responses to manual hyperinflation in post-operative coronary artery surgery patients Physiotherapy Theory and Practice 14 (1998), 5-12.

82. Patman S, Jenkins S, Smith K. Manual hyperinflation: Consistency and modification of the technique by physiotherapists Physiotherapy Research International 6 (2001), 106-17.

83. Patman S, Jenkins S, Stiller K. Manual hyperinflation—effects on respiratory parameters Physiotherapy Research International 5 (2000) 157-71.

84. Pearson SJ. Peak airway pressures exerted during manual hyperinflation by physiotherapists and nursing staff British Journal of Therapy and Rehabilitation 3 (1996), 261-66.

85. Redfern J, Ellis E, Holmes W. The use of a pressure manometer enhances student physiotherapists' performance during manual hyperinflation Australian Journal of Physiotherapy 47 (2001), 121-31.

86. Singer M, Vermaat J, Hall G, Latter G, Patel M. Hemodynamic effects of manual hyperinflation in critically ill mechanically ventilated patients Chest 106 (1994), 1182-87

87. Windsor HM, Harrison GA, Nicholson TJ. 'Bag squeezing': A physiotherapeutic technique Medical Journal of Australia 2 (1972), 829-32.

88. Berney S1, Denehy L, Pretto J. Head-down tilt and manual hyperinflation enhance sputum clearance in patients who are intubated and ventilated. Aust J Physiother 2004;50(1):9-14.

Index